Praise for *Epilepsy*

"This book is an essential guide for people with epilepsy and their families, as well as health care professionals, offering clear, practical insights into understanding and managing the condition. With a thoughtful blend of medical expertise and real-life experiences, it provides readers with the tools to navigate the complexities of epilepsy while fostering hope and empowerment. Whether you're newly diagnosed or have been living with epilepsy for years, this resource will prove invaluable for improving quality of life and supporting informed decisions."

IMAD NAJM, Director, Epilepsy Center and Vice Chair, Neurological Institute, Cleveland Clinic, US

"As someone personally connected to the condition, having suffered from it since a young age, I found this book resonated deeply with me. Beyond the medical explanations, it addresses the emotional and psychological impacts of epilepsy, both from patients and their families. The inclusion of real-life stories added a personal touch, making the book feel relatable and touching. Epilepsy is a must-read for patients, caregivers, and even health care professionals. It offers a blend of expertise, empathy, and practical advice that makes it a standout in the field of medical literature. I highly recommend it for anyone seeking to understand and support those affected by epilepsy."

KATIE COOKE, Young adult, Ireland

"*Epilepsy* provides a clear yet precise description of a complex medical condition that many people are reluctant to discuss. It enhances understanding, particularly of epileptic seizures, and provides an in-depth examination of the causes, how epilepsy is diagnosed, and how it is managed, not only in terms of treatment but also in everyday life. This book will help answer the questions that parents, relatives, and patients have about epilepsy. By offering knowledge and understanding, this well-illustrated book demystifies the condition and aims to empower those affected, bringing hope for a brighter future."

MARIE-CÉCILE NASSOGNE, Head of Pediatric Neurology, Cliniques Universitaires Saint-Luc; Professor, UCLouvain, Belgium

"When a child is diagnosed with epilepsy, a parent may only understand a very limited amount of the information when presented with this overwhelming news. This book is an excellent resource in bridging this gap. It is concise and it presents information in small digestible pieces which are easily comprehensible."

CESAR C. SANTOS, Medical Director, Neurology and Neurosciences, Valley Children's Healthcare, US

"This book is an invaluable resource for anyone seeking to comprehend the complexities of epilepsy, including patients, families, health care students, and professionals not specialized in neurology. It provides a comprehensive yet accessible exploration of epilepsy's diverse presentations, diagnostic challenges, treatment options, and prognostic considerations. What sets this book apart is its compelling integration of case histories, shared by patients and families, which vividly illustrate their journeys through illness and interactions with health care systems. These narratives reveal the triumphs and trials of living with epilepsy, lending a deeply human dimension to the medical insights provided. They are particularly impactful in highlighting the importance of empathy and patient-centred care, making this text a standout resource in an often overly clinical landscape. For patients and families, the book offers both practical information and hope. For health care students, it serves as a vital reminder of the value of the patient voice in shaping compassionate care. It should be required reading for anyone in health care education."

COLIN P. DOHERTY, Head of School of Medicine and Ellen Mayston Bates Chair of Epileptology, Trinity College Dublin, Ireland

"Finally! A book that truly helps families understand epilepsy. As a mother of a special needs child with epilepsy, I found *Epilepsy* to be an invaluable resource. This book skillfully combines medical insights with heartfelt stories, addressing the real-life challenges families like ours face every day. While it offers the depth of a textbook, its clear and accessible writing makes it ideal for parents, caregivers, and educators alike. It provides readers with the knowledge to better understand epilepsy and the confidence to support their loved one. I wish I had this book at the beginning of my journey. It's a must-read for any family navigating life with epilepsy."

COLLEEN PETERSON, parent of son with Wolf-Hirshhorn and Lennox-Gastaut syndromes, US

"This unique book, dedicated to patients and their families, is a simple yet complete explanation of the complex world of epilepsy. Informed discussion and effective communication are key to working out the right treatment for the right patients at the right time. This book goes beyond relaying information; it involves comfort, guidance, and knowledgeable support and trust—the art of care."

MARIA ROBERTA CILIO, MD, PhD, Professor of Pediatric Neurology and Epilepsy, Catholic University of Louvain, Belgium

"*Epilepsy* covers the full range of care for this disorder in easy-to-access language. It is of interest to readers both new and expert in the condition, and points to resources to dive deeper. But the truly unique aspect of this book is the inclusion of vignettes about real patients and their families. Readers can find knowledge to guide them as well as comfort in learning that they are not alone."

ERIK C. BROWN, Pediatric Neurosurgeon, Epilepsy Surgeon, Valley Children's Hospital, US

"Parents and families often lack knowledge of epilepsy and treatment options, and they struggle to find reliable educational resources on this unpredictable disease. This book is an excellent compendium and a comprehensive resource for families with children living with epilepsy. It is a valuable contribution in the service of the epilepsy community and caregivers."

AJAY GUPTA, Head, Pediatric Epilepsy, Cleveland Clinic; Professor, Department of Neurology, Cleveland Clinic Lerner College of Medicine, US

"What makes this book unique is the philosophy behind it. It has a heartfelt, empathic tone, and it beautifully bridges the expertise of pediatric epileptologists with the experiences of families. It empowers doctors by enhancing their ability to explain technical medical terms to patients. The book flows like a story, full of wisdom, knowledge, and hope. It's a must-read for anyone seeking to understand and support individuals affected by epilepsy."

NAEEM MAHFOOZ, Pediatric Neurologist and Epileptologist, ProMedica Neurosciences Center; Associate Professor, University of Toledo, US

"This book provides an exceptional, comprehensive exploration of epilepsy, offering a well-researched, insightful perspective that makes it an invaluable resource for medical professionals, patients and their families, and the general public. One of its standout features is its ability to bridge the gap between the clinical and personal aspects of epilepsy. Through patient and family stories, the authors bring the science to life, offering readers a relatable and compassionate connection to the material. These narratives not only humanize the condition but also help demystify epilepsy, fostering empathy and understanding."

SHANNON GREENE, Surgical Neurophysiologist, US

"A very well written and complete review for health care professionals, which will definitively help clinicians to optimize care for patients with epilepsy. The book is a great summary and guide for patients and their caregivers."

RIËM EL TAHRY, Neurologist and Epileptologist, Cliniques Universitaires Saint-Luc; Principal Investigator, Epilepsy and Neurostimulation Lab, UCLouvain, Belgium

EPILEPSY

EPILEPSY

Understanding and
managing the condition:
A practical guide for families

Charbel El Kosseifi, MD
Cheryl Tveit, RN, MSN, CNML
Anna Halderson, Parent

Edited by
Lily Collison, MA, MSc
Elizabeth R. Boyer, PhD
Timothy Feyma, MD
Tom F. Novacheck, MD
GILLETTE CHILDREN'S

Copyright © 2025 Gillette Children's Healthcare Press

All rights reserved. No part of this publication may be reproduced, stored in a retrieval system, or transmitted in any form or by any means, without the prior written consent of Gillette Children's Healthcare Press.

Gillette Children's Healthcare Press
200 University Avenue East
St Paul, MN 55101
www.GilletteChildrensHealthcarePress.org
HealthcarePress@gillettechildrens.com

ISBN 978-1-952181-19-1 (paperback)
ISBN 978-1-952181-20-7 (e-book)
LIBRARY OF CONGRESS CONTROL NUMBER 2024950609

COPYEDITING BY Ruth Wilson
ORIGINAL ILLUSTRATIONS BY Olwyn Roche
COVER AND INTERIOR DESIGN BY Jazmin Welch
PROOFREADING BY Ruth Wilson
INDEX BY Audrey McClellan
TYPESETTING BY Liz Schreiter

Printed by Hobbs the Printers Ltd, Totton, Hampshire, UK

For information about distribution or special discounts for bulk purchases, please contact:
Mac Keith Press
2nd Floor, Rankin Building
139-143 Bermondsey Street
London, SE1 3UW
www.mackeith.co.uk
admin@mackeith.co.uk

The views and opinions expressed herein are those of the authors and Gillette Children's Healthcare Press and do not necessarily represent those of Mac Keith Press.

To individuals and families whose lives are affected by these conditions, to professionals who serve our community, and to all clinicians and researchers who push the knowledge base forward, we hope the books in this Healthcare Series serve you very well.

All proceeds from the books in this series at Gillette Children's go to research.

All information contained in this book is for educational purposes only. For specific medical advice and treatment, please consult a qualified health care professional. The information in this book is not intended as a substitute for consultation with your health care professional.

Contents

Authors and Editors xv

Series Foreword by Dr. Tom F. Novacheck xvii

Series Introduction xix

1 **SEIZURES AND EPILEPSY: AN OVERVIEW** 1
    1.1   Introduction 3
    1.2   Causes, risk factors, and prevalence 7
    1.3   Seizure first aid 12
    1.4   Differential diagnosis of a seizure 15
    Key points Chapter 1 24

2 **UNDERSTANDING SEIZURES AND EPILEPSY** 25
    2.1   Introduction 27
    2.2   A first seizure: Provoked or unprovoked? 28
    2.3   Classification of seizures 31
    2.4   Phases of a seizure 41
    2.5   Classification of epilepsy 43
    2.6   Overview of epilepsy management 48
    2.7   Sudden unexpected death in epilepsy 53
    Key points Chapter 2 55

3 **THE NERVOUS SYSTEM** 57
    3.1   Introduction 59
    3.2   The brain 61
    3.3   Neurons 70
    3.4   Seizure threshold 73
    Key points Chapter 3 75

4 **EEG AND SEIZURE DETECTION** 77
    WITH ABIGAIL CARLSON, BS, R EEG/EP T, CNIM, NA-CLTM

    4.1   Introduction to EEG 79
    4.2   What happens during EEG? 80

4.3	Interpreting the EEG recording	86
4.4	Phases of a seizure and EEG	92
4.5	Seizure recording and detection	95
	Key points Chapter 4	102

5 DIAGNOSIS OF EPILEPSY 103

5.1	Introduction	105
5.2	Brain imaging	106
5.3	Laboratory tests	108
5.4	Lumbar puncture	112
5.5	Genetic testing	114
	Key points Chapter 5	117

6 CAUSES OF EPILEPSY 119

6.1	Introduction	121
6.2	Structural	123
6.3	Genetic	125
6.4	Infectious	127
6.5	Metabolic	129
6.6	Immune	131
6.7	Unknown	133
	Key points Chapter 6	135

7 EPILEPSY SYNDROMES 137

7.1	Introduction	139
7.2	Onset in the neonatal period and infancy	142
7.3	Onset in childhood	149
7.4	Onset in adolescence and adulthood	154
7.5	Onset at a variable age	157
	Key points Chapter 7	159

8 MANAGEMENT OF EPILEPSY 161

8.1	Introduction	163
8.2	Pharmaceutical management	168
8.3	Non-pharmaceutical management	182
	WITH KARRI LARSON, RD, LD	
8.4	Other medications or supplements	199
8.5	Alternative and complementary therapies	205
	Key points Chapter 8	209

9 COMORBIDITIES OF EPILEPSY 211

    9.1   Introduction 213
    9.2   Neurological and neurodevelopmental comorbidities 216
    9.3   Physical comorbidities 224
    9.4   Psychiatric comorbidities 229
    Key points Chapter 9 232

10 GROWING UP WITH EPILEPSY 233

    10.1   Introduction 235
    10.2   Psychosocial impact of epilepsy 236
    10.3   Activity modifications and lifestyle considerations 238
    10.4   Education and career planning 245
    10.5   Transition to adult care 249
           WITH TORI BAHR, MD
    10.6   Family planning and pregnancy 253
    Key points Chapter 10 258

11 LIVING WITH EPILEPSY 261

12 FURTHER READING AND RESEARCH 287
    WITH ELIZABETH R. BOYER, PhD

Acknowledgments 297

APPENDICES (ONLINE)

    Appendix 1: A short history of epilepsy
    Appendix 2: Seizure mimics
    Appendix 3: Seizure and epilepsy terminology
    Appendix 4: Neurons and seizures
    Appendix 5: Genetic testing and epilepsy
    Appendix 6: Epilepsy syndromes
    Appendix 7: Mechanism of action of antiseizure medications

Glossary 299

References 311

Index 337

Authors and Editors

Charbel El Kosseifi, MD, Pediatric Neurologist and Epileptologist, Gillette Children's

Cheryl Tveit, RN, MSN, CNML, Principal Writer, Gillette Children's Healthcare Press

Anna Halderson, Parent

Lily Collison, MA, MSc, Program Director, Gillette Children's Healthcare Press

Elizabeth R. Boyer, PhD, Clinical Scientist, Gillette Children's

Timothy Feyma, MD, Pediatric Neurologist, Gillette Children's

Tom F. Novacheck, MD, Medical Director of Integrated Care Services, Gillette Children's; Professor of Orthopedics, University of Minnesota; and Past President, American Academy for Cerebral Palsy and Developmental Medicine

Series Foreword

You hold in your hands one book in the Gillette Children's Healthcare Series. This series was inspired by multiple factors.

It started with Lily Collison writing the first book in the series, *Spastic Diplegia–Bilateral Cerebral Palsy*. Lily has a background in medical science and is the parent of a now adult son who has spastic diplegia. Lily was convincing at the time about the value of such a book, and with the publication of that book in 2020, Gillette Children's became one of the first children's hospital in the world to set up its own publishing arm—Gillette Children's Healthcare Press. *Spastic Diplegia–Bilateral Cerebral Palsy* received very positive reviews from both families and professionals and achieved strong sales. Unsolicited requests came in from diverse organizations across the globe for translation rights, and feedback from families told us there was a demand for books relevant to other conditions.

We listened.

We were convinced of the value of expanding from one book into a series to reflect Gillette Children's strong commitment to worldwide education. In 2021, Lily joined the press as Program Director, and very quickly, Gillette Children's formed teams to write the Healthcare Series. The series includes, in order of publication:

- *Craniosynostosis*
- *Idiopathic Scoliosis*
- *Spastic Hemiplegia—Unilateral Cerebral Palsy*
- *Spastic Quadriplegia—Bilateral Cerebral Palsy*
- *Spastic Diplegia—Bilateral Cerebral Palsy, second edition*
- *Epilepsy*
- *Spina Bifida*
- *Osteogenesis Imperfecta*
- *Scoliosis—Congenital, Neuromuscular, Syndromic, and Other Causes*

The books address each condition detailing both the medical and human story.

Mac Keith Press, long-time publisher of books on disability and the journal *Developmental Medicine and Child Neurology*, is co-publishing this series with Gillette Children's Healthcare Press.

Families and professionals working well together is key to best management of any condition. The parent is the expert of their child while the professional is the expert of the condition. These books underscore the importance of that family and professional partnership. For each title in the series, medical professionals at Gillette Children's have led the writing, and families contributed the lived experience.

These books have been written in the United States with an international lens and citing international research. However, there isn't always strong evidence to create consensus in medicine, so others may take a different view.

We hope you find the book you hold in your hands to be of great value. We collectively strive to optimize outcomes for children, adolescents, and adults living with these childhood-acquired and largely lifelong conditions.

Dr. Tom F. Novacheck

Series Introduction

The Healthcare Series seeks to optimize outcomes for those who live with childhood-acquired physical and/or neurological conditions. The conditions addressed in this series of books are complex and often have many associated challenges. Although the books focus on the biomedical aspects of each condition, we endeavor to address each condition as holistically as possible. Since the majority of people with these conditions have them for life, the life course is addressed including transition and aging issues.

Who are these books for?

These books are written for an international audience. They are primarily written for parents of young children, but also for adolescents and adults who have the condition. They are written for members of multidisciplinary teams and researchers. Finally, they are written for others, including extended family members, teachers, and students taking courses in the fields of medicine, allied health care, and education.

A worldview

The books in the series focus on evidence-based best practice, which we acknowledge is not available everywhere. It is mostly available in high-income countries (at least in urban areas, though even there, not always), but many families live away from centers of good care.

We also acknowledge that the majority of people with disabilities live in low- and middle-income countries. Improving the lives of all those with disabilities across the globe is an important goal. Developing scalable, affordable interventions is a crucial step toward achieving this. Nonetheless, the best interventions will fail if we do not first address the social determinants of health—the economic, social, and environmental conditions in which people live that shape their overall health and well-being.

No family reading these books should ever feel they have failed their child. We all struggle to do our best for our children within the limitations of our various resources and situations. Indeed, the advocacy role these books may play may help families and professionals lobby in unison for best care.

International Classification of Functioning, Disability and Health

The writing of the series of books has been informed by the International Classification of Functioning, Disability and Health (ICF).[1] The framework explains the impact of a health condition at different levels and how those levels are interconnected. It tells us to look at the full picture—to look at the person with a disability in their life situation.

The framework shows that every human being can experience a decrease in health and thereby experience some disability. It is not something that happens only to a minority of people. The ICF thus "mainstreams" disability and recognizes it as a widespread human experience.

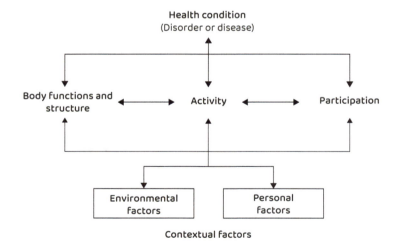

International Classification of Functioning, Disability and Health (ICF). Reproduced with kind permission from WHO.

In health care, there has been a shift away from focusing almost exclusively on correcting issues that cause the individual's functional problems to focusing also on the individual's activity and participation. These books embrace maximizing participation for all people living with disability.

The family

For simplicity, throughout the series we refer to "parents" and "children"; we acknowledge, however, that family structures vary. "Parent" is used as a generic term that includes grandparents, relatives, and carers (caregivers) who are raising a child. Throughout the series, we refer to male and female as the biologic sex assigned at birth. We acknowledge that this does not equate to gender identity or sexual orientation, and we respect the individuality of each person. Throughout the series we have included both "person with disability" and "disabled person," recognizing that both terms are used.

Caring for a child with a disability can be challenging and overwhelming. Having a strong social support system in place can make a difference. For the parent, balancing the needs of the child with a disability with the needs of siblings—while also meeting employment demands, nurturing a relationship with a significant other, and caring for aging parents—can sometimes feel like an enormous juggling act. Siblings may feel neglected or overlooked because of the increased attention given to the disabled child. It is crucial for parents to allocate time and resources to ensure that siblings feel valued and included in the family dynamics. Engaging siblings in the care and support of the disabled child can help foster a sense of unity and empathy within the family.

A particular challenge for a child and adolescent who has a disability, and their parent, is balancing school attendance (for both academic and social purposes) with clinical appointments and surgery. Appointments outside of school hours are encouraged. School is important because the cognitive and social abilities developed there help maximize employment opportunities when employment is a realistic goal. Indeed, technology has eliminated barriers and created opportunities that did not exist even 10 years ago.

Parents also need to find a way to prioritize self-care. Neglecting their own well-being can have detrimental effects on their mental and physical health. Think of the safety advice on an airplane: you are told that you must put on your own oxygen mask before putting on your child's. It's the same when caring for a child with a disability; parents need to take care of themselves in order to effectively care for their child and family. Friends, support groups, or mental health professionals can provide an outlet for parents to express their emotions, gain valuable insights, and find solace in knowing that they are not alone in their journey.

For those of you reading this book who have the condition, we hope this book gives you insights into its many nuances and complexities, acknowledges you as the expert in your own care and provides a road map and framework for you to advocate for your needs.

Last words

This series of books seeks to be an invaluable educational resource. All proceeds from the series at Gillette Children's go to research.

Chapter 1

Seizures and epilepsy:
An overview

Section 1.1 Introduction 3
Section 1.2 Causes, risk factors, and prevalence 7
Section 1.3 Seizure first aid 12
Section 1.4 Differential diagnosis of a seizure 15
Key points Chapter 1 24

1.1 Introduction

> Nothing in life is to be feared,
> it is only to be understood.
> Now is the time to understand more,
> so that we may fear less.
> **Marie Curie**

A seizure is an unexpected event that occurs suddenly, and experiencing or witnessing it can be scary and create helpless feelings. Having an understanding of seizures and epilepsy can help you feel more in control of the situation. While epilepsy can occur at any age, the focus of this book is primarily on epilepsy that begins in the time before adulthood—that is, during infancy, childhood, or adolescence.

If you are reading this as a parent of a child with a diagnosis of seizures or epilepsy, or you are an individual who is affected by seizures or epilepsy, these terms are likely familiar. "Seizure" and "epilepsy" are sometimes used interchangeably, but in fact, they are distinct terms with different meanings.

The definition of "seizure" is "uncontrolled, abnormal electrical activity of the brain that may cause changes in the level of consciousness, behavior, memory, or feelings."[2] The abnormal electrical activity of a seizure may result in a change in the individual's consciousness, physical movement, behavior, sensation, or feelings that can be brief or long-lasting.[3] A seizure may be obvious to an observer, and it may include jerking, shaking, twisting, or other physical movements. Some seizures occur without any outward physical signs but are accompanied by feelings or sensations experienced by the individual having the seizure.

While a seizure is an isolated event, epilepsy is a condition often characterized by *recurrent, unprovoked* seizures.[4] The term "unprovoked" in the context of seizures describes a seizure that occurs without a specific acute cause. "Acute" means occurring with an abrupt onset.

The most widely accepted definition of epilepsy, developed by the International League Against Epilepsy (ILAE), is a condition affecting an individual who has any of the following:[5,6]

1. **"At least two unprovoked (or reflex) seizures occurring more than 24 hours apart"**: While epilepsy is typically characterized by *unprovoked* seizures, a reflex seizure is one type of *provoked* seizure that consistently occurs in response to a stimulus, such as light or reading, and may be classified as epilepsy.
2. **"One unprovoked (or reflex) seizure and a probability of further seizures similar to the general recurrence risk (at least 60%) after two unprovoked seizures, occurring over the next 10 years"**: In other words, epilepsy is diagnosed if the individual has the same chance of having a second seizure over the next 10 years as someone who already has had two *unprovoked* seizures. Therefore, the epilepsy diagnosis may be made even if an individual has had only one seizure.
3. **"Diagnosis of an epilepsy syndrome"**: A syndrome is a group of characteristics that consistently occur together. An epilepsy syndrome is "a characteristic cluster of clinical and EEG features, often supported by specific etiological findings (structural, genetic,

metabolic, immune, and infectious)."*7 In very rare cases, an individual may be diagnosed with an epilepsy syndrome without experiencing any seizures.

Not all seizures lead to a diagnosis of epilepsy. *However, an epileptic seizure is a seizure associated with a diagnosis of epilepsy.*

The ILAE is a resource of best practice for medical professionals, patients, care providers, governments, and the public on the care of individuals with epilepsy. Definitions, classifications, and guidelines developed by the ILAE (www.ilae.org) are referenced throughout this book.

How to read this book

The aim of this book is to allow you to learn about seizures and epilepsy at your own pace. For some individuals, epilepsy will be a lifelong, chronic condition, while for others it may be something they outgrow. Epilepsy may have a large impact on an individual's daily life, requiring multiple management techniques, or it may be well controlled and have little daily impact other than having to remember to take medication. The span of possibilities with an epilepsy diagnosis is broad.

The information presented in this book may feel overwhelming, and not all aspects covered will be relevant to all individuals. Though you can read each chapter in this book independently, much of the information builds on information in previous chapters, so it is best to first read the book in its entirety to get an overall sense of the condition. After that, sections not currently relevant to you can be ignored and revisited if or when they become pertinent.

Throughout, medical information is interspersed with the personal lived experience of Anna Halderson, who writes about her family's journey navigating the epilepsy diagnosis of her daughter, Emma. Orange-colored boxes highlight their personal story. Chapter 11 is devoted to vignettes from other individuals and families around the globe. At the back of the book, you'll find a glossary of key terms.

---

* Key terms in this definition: "EEG" (electroencephalography measures the brain's electrical activity); "etiological" (relating to the cause); "metabolic" (referring to chemical processes that help cells in the body convert food into energy).

A companion website with appendices for this book is available at www.GilletteChildrensHealthcarePress.org. A QR code to access **Useful web resources** is included below.

While this book is forward looking, a short history of epilepsy is included in Appendix 1 (online).

It may be helpful to discuss any questions you may have from reading this book with your medical professional.

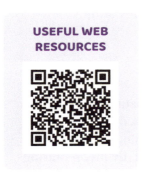

1.2 Causes, risk factors, and prevalence

> The measure of who we are is
> what we do with what we have.
> Vince Lombardi

Causes of seizures

Seizures may be either provoked or unprovoked, and each type has different causes.

a) Provoked seizures

A provoked seizure, also called an acute symptomatic seizure, is a seizure associated with a systemic (throughout the body) injury or a brain injury. A provoked seizure usually occurs as a single seizure and does not lead to a diagnosis of epilepsy. An exception is a reflex seizure, which is one type of provoked seizure included in the definition of epilepsy.[8] Reflex seizures occur after a particular stimulus, are very rare, and are typically associated with a reflex epilepsy syndrome (e.g., reading epilepsy and startle epilepsy).

Causes of provoked seizures include (but are not limited to):[2,3]

- Fever
- Gastroenteritis
- Infection or inflammation in the brain or spinal cord, such as meningitis or encephalitis
- Electrolyte imbalance with or without dehydration (Electrolytes include iron, calcium, magnesium, potassium, and other minerals.)
- Brain injury
- Brain tumor
- Stroke
- Cardiac abnormalities (e.g., arrythmias, which are atypical heart rhythms that may be too slow, too fast, or irregular)
- Illicit drug use*
- Alcohol withdrawal
- Rarely, stimuli such as flashing lights, hyperventilation (rapid breathing), reading, or listening to a certain type of music

Two common types of provoked seizures in infants and children that often resolve without treatment are febrile seizures and benign convulsions associated with mild gastroenteritis:

- **Febrile seizures:** These occur in infants and children between the ages of six months and five years and are associated with a temperature of at least 100.4 °F (38 °C) without brain or spinal cord infection.[9] Febrile seizures often occur along with viral illnesses.[10] In Western countries, 2 to 5 percent of young children experience febrile seizures.[10] Once a child experiences a febrile seizure, they are at a higher risk of having another: approximately one in three children will have a second febrile seizure.[9,11] Children experiencing *simple* febrile seizures (lasting less than 15 minutes and not recurring within 24 hours) have only a slightly increased risk of developing epilepsy (1 to 2 percent) as a child without febrile seizures (0.5 percent).[9] Children experiencing *complex* febrile seizures (lasting longer than 15 minutes, or recurring within 24 hours, or occurring

---

* "Illicit drug use" refers to using and misusing both illegal and controlled drugs. Withdrawing from illicit drugs may also lead to seizures and should be coordinated under the care of a medical professional.

only on one side or area of the body) have an increased risk of developing epilepsy (6 to 8 percent).[9]
- **Benign convulsions associated with mild gastroenteritis:** The term "benign" means not harmful.[*] Convulsions are involuntary, uncontrolled muscle contractions that cause motor (movement) activity and may occur during a seizure.[12,13] Gastroenteritis is a condition that causes inflammation and irritation of the digestive system leading to vomiting, diarrhea, or nausea. Benign convulsions associated with mild gastroenteritis occur in infants and children age 2 months to 6 years, peaking between 12 and 24 months.[14] Seizures usually occur within six days of the onset of diarrhea and typically resolve on their own within a few days. These seizures typically do not recur.[14]

b) Unprovoked seizures

Recurrent, unprovoked seizures are associated with a diagnosis of epilepsy. Causes of unprovoked seizures that lead to a diagnosis of epilepsy include:[15]

- A structural abnormality of the brain
- A genetic abnormality, closely associated with pathologic changes in genes[†16]
- A previous (not acute) infection in the brain
- A metabolic[‡] disorder
- An immune disorder (an alteration in the body's defense system against infections)
- Unknown

Note that the causes of unprovoked seizures are also the causes of epilepsy, which are described in Chapter 6.

---

[*] For most individuals, benign convulsions associated with mild gastroenteritis resolve on their own, but some individuals who have additional medical conditions may require additional monitoring and treatment.

[†] Genes are the units of heredity transferred from parent to offspring. Genetics is a branch of science that studies genes or heredity.

[‡] "Metabolic" refers to chemical processes that allow cells in the body to convert food into energy, clean up cellular waste products, or impact the many chemical reactions involved in the life cycle of cells.

Risk factors for developing seizures and epilepsy

The term "risk factor" is defined as "an aspect of personal behavior or lifestyle, an environmental exposure, or an inborn or inherited characteristic that is associated with an increased occurrence of disease or other health-related event or condition."[17]

Certain risk factors may make it more likely that someone will have a seizure, but not all seizures will be diagnosed as epilepsy. Specific risk factors for developing seizures and epilepsy include (but are not limited to):[18]

- Family history of seizures
- Select genetic disorders
- Infants born small for age or premature
- Infants with atypical brain structure or development
- Complex febrile seizures[9]
- Brain injury, bleeding, or lack of oxygen
- Cerebral palsy*
- Brain tumors
- Infections of the brain
- Atypical blood vessels in the brain or a stroke resulting from blockage of arteries (blood vessels carrying blood from the heart to areas of the body)
- Late-stage Alzheimer's disease
- Autism spectrum disorder
- Age (young children and older adults are at the highest risk)[19]

Prevalence of seizures and epilepsy

"Prevalence" means the proportion of a population with a specific characteristic or condition in a specified period, often expressed as a percentage. Prevalence of a condition fluctuates depending on screening and identification of new cases, availability of curative treatments, and overall life expectancy of individuals with the condition.[20] When

---

* Cerebral palsy (CP) is a group of permanent disorders of the development of movement and posture, caused by a brain injury during pregnancy or shortly after birth.

considering the prevalence of seizures and epilepsy, it is important to note some distinctions:

- Anyone can have a seizure at any point in their lifetime.
- Seizures are more common than epilepsy.
- Up to 10 percent of people will have one seizure in their lifetime, while only 0.8 to 3.8 percent will develop epilepsy in their lifetime.[19,21,22]

Epilepsy occurs across the world in all ages, races, and social classes.[23] Disparities exist, however.

- The World Health Organization estimates that over 50 million people worldwide are living with epilepsy, and nearly 80 percent reside in low- and middle-income countries and have less access to antiseizure medications.[21,24] (Antiseizure medications are medications that work to *prevent, reduce*, or *stop* seizures).
- In low- and middle-income countries, the incidence of childhood epilepsy is three times higher than in high-income countries.[25] The lack of resources to prevent and treat infections as well as higher rates of injuries are likely contributors to this disparity.[25] Prevention of epilepsy is believed to be possible in approximately 25 percent of cases.[24]

The prevalence of epilepsy is increasing, likely because more people are surviving events such as serious head trauma, strokes, brain tumors, and brain infections,[21,22] and because life expectancy is increasing worldwide (older people are at increased risk for epilepsy).[22,24]

1.3 Seizure first aid

Confidence comes from being prepared.
John Wooden

Witnessing someone having a seizure can be scary. Understanding seizure first aid can help individuals and their caregivers to remain calm. Individuals who experience seizures, or their caregivers, should share first aid information with people close to them—teachers, coworkers, friends, and others—so everyone is knowledgeable about seizure first aid and can respond to a seizure appropriately.

The Epilepsy Foundation has developed the code STAY, SAFE, SIDE* as a quick way to remember seizure first aid[26] (see Figure 1.3.1).

---

* Turning an individual on their side during a seizure is recommended to help prevent aspiration from occurring. However, do not restrain or restrict movement of an individual who is actively seizing.

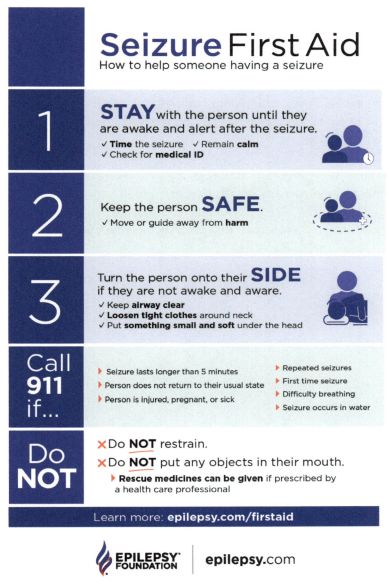

Figure 1.3.1 Seizure first aid poster. Reproduced from the Epilepsy Foundation © 2024. Note that 911 is the standard emergency number in the US; other countries have their own emergency telephone numbers. Medical IDs are cards or wearable items that contain health information about the individual that may be helpful for first responders.

After a first seizure or a suspected seizure occurs, the individual should be seen by a medical professional as soon as possible. A thorough medical history and physical examination will be done to determine:

- Whether or not the event is a seizure
- If an acute cause can be identified
- If the event is classified as a seizure, whether the seizure is provoked or unprovoked

When possible, parents, caregivers, or onlookers should record the event and write down any details to share with the medical professional.

Further information on seizure first aid is included in **Useful web resources.**

1.4 Differential diagnosis of a seizure

> Not I, nor anyone else can travel that road for you.
> You must travel it by yourself.
> It is not far, it is within reach.
> Perhaps you have been on it since you were born and did not know.
> Perhaps it is everywhere—on water on land.
> **Walt Whitman**

The term "differential diagnosis" is used to refer to the list of potential medical conditions that could explain an individual's symptoms. It also describes the meticulous process of eliminating other possible causes to arrive at a medical diagnosis. This process is frequently used in the diagnosis of seizures and epilepsy.

Not all events that look like a seizure are in fact a seizure. A seizure is often obvious, but sometimes an event characterized by a change in consciousness, physical movement, behavior, sensation, or feeling appears to be a seizure but is not; rather, it is due to another condition. This is referred to as a "seizure mimic" or a "nonepileptic event." To differentiate between them, the medical professional uses the process of differential diagnosis to decide if the event is a seizure or a seizure mimic. Meticulously eliminating seizure mimics is done before diagnosing the event as a seizure.

Close evaluation of both the circumstances around the event and the characteristics of the individual may be enough to diagnose the event as a seizure. Circumstances and characteristics evaluated may include sounds, presence of triggers, duration of the event, fever, movements, posture, level of consciousness, and emotions. For example, when a child experiences an event that appears like a seizure and has a viral illness with a fever over 100.4 °F (38 °C) but no brain or spinal cord infection, then the event may be quickly diagnosed as a febrile seizure.

Some seizure mimics are more common in certain age groups, which is helpful information during the process of differential diagnosis. Referrals to specialists and additional testing, such as EEG (electroencephalography, to measure the brain's electrical activity) may also be needed to make a diagnosis.

Common seizure mimics are presented below by the age group in which they most often occur or start to be noticed. This list is not exhaustive.

Seizure mimics in the neonatal period and infancy

A neonate is a child less than four weeks of age, and an infant is a child under one year of age.[27,28] Seizure mimics that may occur in the neonatal period and infancy include the following:

- **Gastroesophageal reflux disease:** GERD—or acid reflux—is a condition where liquid contents from the stomach go back into the esophagus.[29] In a neonate or infant, this causes irritability, excessive crying, sleep disturbances, and muscle contractions.[30]
- **Sandifer syndrome:** This movement disorder involves involuntary muscle contractions, back arching, stiffening of the neck, and turning or tilting the head. It often occurs along with GERD, typically within 30 minutes of feeding.[31-33]
- **Breath-holding spell:** A breath-holding spell is triggered by a vigorous crying episode after which the child holds their breath (as a reflex, not on purpose). It may be accompanied by body stiffness or

convulsions and may occur along with loss of consciousness and cyanosis (bluish skin coloring) or paleness.[31,34]
- **Benign spasms of infancy:** The term "benign" means something that is not harmful. "Spasms" are brief, involuntary muscle contractions. Benign spasms of infancy include rapid movements of the head, trunk, and shoulders with brief jerking of limbs on both sides.[35] This condition occurs in infants and resolves on its own in the second year of life.[35]

Successful treatment of the seizure mimic, such as with gastric protection medication for GERD, may help differentiate a seizure mimic from a seizure.[30] If it is unclear whether the event is triggered by GERD or is a seizure, the child may be referred to a gastroenterologist,[*] and gastrointestinal tests may be recommended. If a breath-holding spell appears to be cardiac in nature, a referral to a cardiologist[†] may be recommended.[34] Benign spasms of infancy may be differentiated from seizures by EEG.[35]

Seizure mimics in childhood

"Childhood" is defined as being the period between infancy and adolescence—age one to nine years. The following are seizure mimics that may occur during childhood:

- **Cyclic vomiting:** A condition that includes repeated bouts of vomiting often accompanied by abdominal pain, pallor (pale skin coloring), fatigue, and may also occur along with migraine headaches.[31] Vomiting often occurs in a very predictable pattern and will last for a certain number of days and then resolve.[31]
- **Hypoglycemia:** A condition with lower than typical blood glucose (sugar) levels, resulting in confusion, a loss of or decrease in consciousness, lack of coordination, difficulties with speech, and tremors.[36,37]

---

[*] A gastroenterologist is a medical professional who specializes in the care of the digestive system, including the stomach and intestines.

[†] A cardiologist is a medical professional who specializes in the care of the heart and blood vessels.

- **Migraine:** A type of headache with moderate to severe throbbing and pulsating pain. These often recur, and the pain may be concentrated on one side of the head.[38] Migraines may be accompanied by an aura (a sensation or symptom experienced at the onset of a neurological event including sudden intense feelings of fear or joy, a feeling of déjà vu, numbness or tingling, unusual tastes or smells, visual disturbances, feeling dizzy, headaches, or nausea).[39,40]
- **Movement disorders**
  - **Stereotypies:** Semivoluntary repetitive movements that are often rhythmic and may include clapping or arm shaking.[31,41] These are usually not associated with loss of consciousness and may occur multiple times per day.[41]
  - **Tics:** Involuntary, sudden, rapid, and repetitive sounds or movements. Vocal tics may include throat clearing, coughing, grunting, or yelling. Motor tics may include blinking, eye rolling, mouth movements, shaking of hands, tapping, kicking, or abnormal postures.[42]
- **Sleep disorders**
  - **Narcolepsy:** A sleep disorder characterized by excessive sleepiness during the day and often presenting with irresistible sleep attacks.[43] Cataplexy (the loss of postural muscle tone, causing the individual to fall suddenly) is common. Hallucinations or paralysis when falling asleep or when waking may also occur.[37]
  - **Parasomnias:** A group of sleep disorders characterized by unusual behaviors that occur just before falling asleep, while asleep, or just upon waking, and may be accompanied by loss of consciousness and the inability to recall the event.[44-46]
  - **Sleep myoclonus:** A sudden, involuntary muscle jerk often accompanied by a hallucination of movement, experienced as a feeling of falling.[45] These events are very brief and occur during sleep transitions (falling asleep or waking up).[47]

To differentiate seizure mimics from seizures in a child, the medical professional may order laboratory tests or other evaluations. For example, if it is unclear whether the child is experiencing cyclic vomiting or a seizure, a referral to a gastroenterologist and additional gastrointestinal tests may be needed.[31] Blood glucose levels may be measured to evaluate for hypoglycemia, or a polysomnogram (sleep study) may be ordered to evaluate for sleep disorders.[36,44] Migraines can be assessed by their aura (if auras occur; migraine auras have a gradual onset compared to seizure auras, which tend to have an abrupt onset).[39,40,44] Tics and stereotypies may be momentarily suppressed by the individual, unlike seizures, which may help in identifying these as seizure mimics.[41,48]

Seizure mimics in adolescence and adulthood

Adolescence is the period between ages 10 and 19 years, and adulthood begins at 19 years.[49] The following are seizure mimics that may occur during adolescence and adulthood:

- **Behavioral, psychological, and psychiatric conditions:** These may include dissociative disorders,[*] panic attacks, hyperventilation, and episodic dyscontrol.[†][50,51] These conditions may be brought on by personal or environmental stressors and typically do not involve a change in consciousness.[32,39,44,51]
- **Cardiovascular conditions:** These involve the heart and vascular system, including heart abnormalities, heart rhythm abnormalities (long QT syndrome),[‡] high blood pressure, or postural orthostatic tachycardia syndrome (POTS).[§][52,53] Individuals experiencing cardiovascular conditions may become pale, limp, or lightheaded; have blurred vision or abdominal pain; and experience syncope or a loss of consciousness.[32,52,53]
- **Cerebrovascular conditions:** These involve the brain and vascular system and include brain abnormalities, strokes, or transient ischemic attacks (TIAs).[¶][54,55] Individuals experiencing cerebrovascular conditions may have difficulty with speech, vision, or lack of movement on one side of the body.[41]

---

* Dissociative disorders are psychiatric conditions that involve disruptions related to memory, identity, emotion, perception, and behavior.

† "Episodic dyscontrol" means recurrent attacks of uncontrollable rage and violence followed by exhaustion and difficulty recalling the event. This is also known as intermittent explosive disorder.

‡ Long QT syndrome is a condition of abnormal heart rhythm that causes syncope (fainting) and may lead to death.

§ POTS is a group of conditions where blood flows to the heart after a change of position, resulting in a symptom known as orthostatic intolerance. Individuals with orthostatic intolerance feel faint or lightheaded when they move from lying to standing.

¶ A stroke is a condition in which a blood vessel in the brain is either blocked or ruptured, damaging the brain and causing symptoms such as paralysis, speech problems, and memory loss. A TIA is a condition in which a blood vessel in the brain is temporarily blocked causing temporary symptoms like a stroke.

- **Psychogenic nonepileptic seizures (PNES):** These involuntary events may last for several minutes (sometimes 15 to 30 minutes or longer) and often involve loss of consciousness or motor signs such as irregular jerking or shaking of the limbs and falling.[32,37,56] PNES is a serious condition that may significantly impact quality of life, and therefore the differentiation of the two is especially important.[57] The term "functional seizure" may be used interchangeably with "PNES."
- **Syncope (fainting spell):** This involves self-limiting,*[58] transient (temporary) loss of consciousness with the inability to maintain a standing or unsupported posture. It may be accompanied by brief jerking movements.[59–61] Sometimes, a cardiovascular condition (e.g., heart rhythm disturbance or atypical structure in the heart) may lead to a syncope event.

Often, seizure mimics in adolescents and adults are triggered by specific events, locations, or emotions.[31] For example, syncope typically occurs only from a standing position, not from a sitting position or while lying down, unlike seizures.[59] It may be triggered by pain, emotions, prolonged standing, or a hot environment and is often preceded by dizziness, nausea, paleness, or sweating.[37,61,62] The individual typically regains consciousness quickly after syncope, unlike with a seizure, where they often feel tired and disoriented, and may experience a slow return to consciousness.[63,64] Behavioral, psychological, and psychiatric conditions are often triggered by school or work problems or social and environmental stressors, which are different than typical seizure triggers.

Differentiating seizure mimics from seizures in adolescents and adults may be done by evaluating triggers, using imaging, or conducting laboratory tests. EEG is typically used to help with differential diagnosis. For differentiating cardiovascular and cerebrovascular conditions, specialized tests may be used, such as echocardiogram (ultrasound of the heart) and ECG (electrocardiogram; recording of the electrical activity of the heart, also called EKG).

More information on seizure mimics can be found in Appendix 2 (online). Figure 1.4.1 summarizes the differential diagnosis of a seizure.

---

* "Self-limiting" means to limit itself or spontaneously resolve.

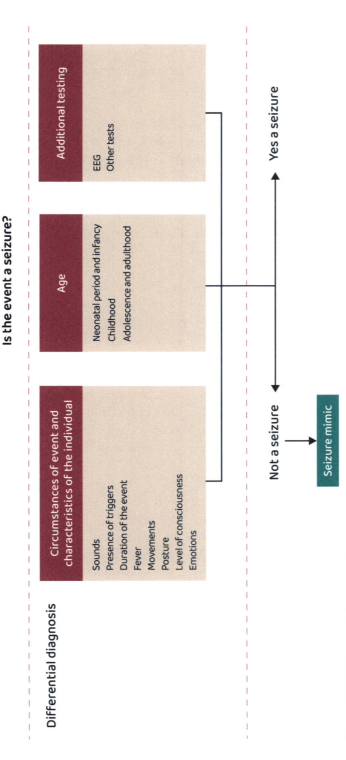

Figure 1.4.1 Differential diagnosis of a seizure.

My husband, Scott, and I live in a small rural town outside of Saint Paul, Minnesota. We are parents to twins, Emma and Jake, who are now young adults, age 20 at the time of writing. Emma has many complex medical conditions, including epilepsy.

In spring 2003, I was a 24-year-old first-time mother. Scott and I had just found out at my 20-week ultrasound that I was carrying twins. Of course, we were surprised and excited all at the same time. We were told we were having a boy and a girl: I had Emma's name picked out for a long time before the birth, while Jake's name was picked just before he was born. Like any expecting mom, I dreamed about the day I would get to hold my babies for the first time. I anxiously looked forward to the birth.

Six weeks later, for reasons still unknown, I spontaneously went into premature labor, delivering our precious twins at only 26 weeks. Emma came first, weighing 1 lb, 12 oz (794 grams), and Jake followed 39 minutes later, weighing 1 lb, 15 oz (879 grams). After they were born, I was so overwhelmed with a lot of mixed feelings and emotions. This was not at all the labor and delivery I had imagined or expected. I was ecstatic that we had been blessed with not just one but two beautiful babies, but we also felt so unprepared. The excitement of being a new mom was immediately overshadowed by a dark cloud of fear and uncertainty. Would the babies survive? What would the future look like? What would happen now?

Those first weeks are a bit of a blur. I recall feeling confused, scared, and worried. When the twins were just two days old, Emma had a CT scan and the doctor sat us down and told us that she had suffered a grade IV intraventricular hemorrhage, explained to us as bleeding on her brain caused by her premature birth. She was also diagnosed with hydrocephalus,* and we learned that she would need to have a shunt† placed. I had a large lump in my throat with that news and felt anyone looking at me could surely see this from the outside—it felt so large.

---

* A condition in which there is a buildup of cerebrospinal fluid (fluid that surrounds the brain and spinal canal) in cavities (ventricles) in the brain.

† A device inserted into the ventricles of the brain; the shunt tubing (catheter) drains the cerebrospinal fluid from the ventricles and transports it to a reservoir where it is stored and then moved to the peritoneal cavity (a space within the abdominal area not occupied by the abdominal organs). There, the fluid is absorbed by the body.

I knew what he was telling us was not good, but I didn't understand what he was saying and, frankly, I felt stupid that I *didn't* have a greater understanding of what was going on. I didn't know all the medical lingo I was hearing, and because all this happened before it was easy to find anything with an Internet search, I relied on my ability to ask the staff a million questions. I tried to look things up in books, but it was so time-consuming and difficult to understand. I felt inadequate and small.

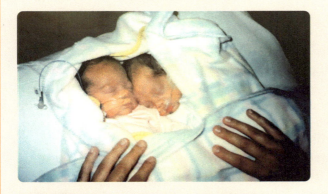

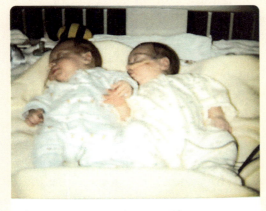

Top: Jake (left) and Emma. Bottom: Emma (left) and Jake in the NICU.

Key points Chapter 1

- The terms "seizure" and "epilepsy" are sometimes used interchangeably, but they are distinct terms with different meanings. Anyone can have a seizure, and up to 10 percent of people will have one seizure in their lifetime. Epilepsy is much less common than seizures and 0.8 to 3.8 percent of people will develop epilepsy.
- A seizure is uncontrolled, abnormal electrical activity of the brain that may cause changes in the level of consciousness, behavior, memories, or feelings. Seizures can be provoked or unprovoked.
- Provoked seizures are due to an acute cause and are usually not associated with epilepsy. Common causes for provoked seizures in infants and children are fever (above 100.4 °F or 38 °C) or gastroenteritis (an acute illness with nausea, vomiting, and diarrhea).
- Unprovoked seizures are not due to an acute cause and are more often associated with epilepsy. Unprovoked seizures can be caused by structural or genetic abnormalities; a brain infection; or metabolic, immune, or unknown disorders.
- Epilepsy is a condition often characterized by recurrent, unprovoked seizures.
- Risk factors for epilepsy include a family history of seizures or epilepsy, a history of brain injury or brain abnormalities, cerebral palsy, and other factors.
- Epilepsy occurs across the world in all ages, races, and social classes. However, nearly 80 percent of individuals with epilepsy live in low- and middle-income countries. The prevalence of epilepsy is increasing due to improved survival rates for serious injuries and increased life expectancy.
- Seizure first aid includes STAY, SAFE, SIDE, providing direction to those who are assisting an individual experiencing a seizure.
- Not all events that look like a seizure are a seizure; some are known as seizure mimics, and differential diagnosis is used to rule out other causes of the events before determining if the individual indeed had a seizure.

Chapter 2

Understanding seizures and epilepsy

Section 2.1 Introduction 27
Section 2.2 A first seizure: Provoked or unprovoked? 28
Section 2.3 Classification of seizures 31
Section 2.4 Phases of a seizure 41
Section 2.5 Classification of epilepsy 43
Section 2.6 Overview of epilepsy management 48
Section 2.7 Sudden unexpected death in epilepsy 53
Key points Chapter 2 55

2.1 Introduction

> The improvement of understanding is for two ends:
> first, our own increase of knowledge; secondly,
> to enable us to deliver that knowledge to others.
> **John Locke**

This chapter describes the process that occurs after a first seizure is diagnosed to determine if the seizure is provoked or unprovoked (section 2.2). Seizures are also classified into types, which is addressed in section 2.3. A seizure occurs in phases, which is addressed in section 2.4. Classification of epilepsy, including epilepsy type, etiology (cause), epilepsy syndrome, and comorbidities, is addressed in section 2.5. While these steps are presented in order, the diagnosis of epilepsy is individualized and does not always follow an exact path.

An overview of managing epilepsy is addressed in section 2.6. Finally, a rare complication of epilepsy known as sudden unexpected death in epilepsy (SUDEP) is addressed in section 2.7.

USEFUL WEB RESOURCES

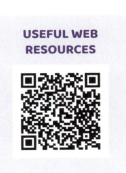

2.2 A first seizure: Provoked or unprovoked?

> Worry is like a rocking chair.
> It will give you something to do
> but never gets you anywhere.
> **Erma Bombeck**

Once established that the event is a seizure, the next step is to determine if it is provoked or unprovoked. This is done by looking for any possible acute cause that would provoke the seizure. The decision tree for determining whether a seizure is provoked is shown in Figure 2.2.1.

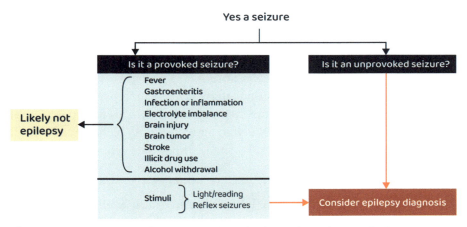

Figure 2.2.1 Decision tree for determining whether seizure is provoked or unprovoked.

An individual who has a first provoked seizure is not likely to have another seizure and is not likely to be diagnosed with epilepsy.[65,66] Once a provoked seizure has been ruled out, the seizure is termed "unprovoked," and the medical professional may consider an epilepsy diagnosis. The next steps will include watching for a second seizure and may involve the following:

- EEG
- Brain imaging (MRI or CT)
- Laboratory tests

While the recurrence of unprovoked seizures is more common than provoked seizures, most people experiencing a single unprovoked seizure (50 to 70 percent) will not ever have a second seizure or be diagnosed with epilepsy.[65] The risk of experiencing a second unprovoked seizure decreases with time:[66]

- 50 percent of second seizures occur within six months of the initial seizure.
- 76 to 96 percent of second seizures occur within two years of the initial seizure.

Recall that epilepsy is a condition typically characterized by *recurrent, unprovoked* seizures. The presence of risk factors for the development of epilepsy (see section 1.2) increases the likelihood that an individual will have a second unprovoked seizure.

The path to diagnosing epilepsy is not always straightforward. In some individuals, a medical professional may suspect epilepsy with the first seizure or when other conditions are present (e.g., cerebral palsy) that may make individuals more likely to have epilepsy. The diagnosis of epilepsy may be quick or may take time, sometimes years.

> As the weeks went by, our son Jake did remarkably well, in stark contrast to how things were going with Emma. They both "graduated" from the NICU and were moved to another unit. I felt hopeful for Emma with the move—feeling it was good news and that things were going to be okay.
>
> I can clearly recall the first time Emma had a seizure. I had stepped out of the new stepdown unit the twins were in to make a phone call and take a break from the nonstop schedule of being a new mom. When I returned, Emma's nurse and a doctor were standing by her crib, and I could tell something was wrong. I felt that awful lump in my throat come back again. I saw Emma moving, but just subtly. The doctor attempted to stop the movement by putting her hands over Emma's arms, but Emma kept moving. At that point, the doctor told me, with hesitation in her voice, that Emma had just had a seizure. My heart sank. I looked at my precious daughter's sweet face and wondered why all this was happening to her. The questions and what-ifs started to flood my mind. Was this whole situation my fault? Had I done something during my pregnancy to cause this? Or had I not done something I should have done? I even wondered if other people were thinking this as well. Maybe it was the diet soda I drank that day at work. Or the fast food I kept craving and made a stop for on my way home from work. Maybe I shouldn't have even been working. Maybe I did too much, or maybe I didn't do enough.

2.3 Classification of seizures

A process cannot be understood by stopping it. Understanding must move with the flow of the process, must join it and flow with it.
Frank Herbert

This section explains the classification of seizures—first, second, and third—and what each is based on:

- First classification: Seizure onset zone
- Second classification: Level of awareness during a seizure
- Third classification: Motor or nonmotor

First classification: Seizure onset zone

A seizure is first classified based on where it begins in the brain, termed the "seizure onset zone" (see Figure 2.3.1):[67] To understand seizure onset zones, it is important to know that the brain is divided into two halves, referred to as hemispheres (right or left). In general, the right hemisphere controls the left side of the body, and the left hemisphere controls the right side of the body. The anatomy of the brain is further described in Chapter 3.

- **Focal onset seizure:** A seizure that starts from one half of the brain. Focal onset seizures lead to signs and symptoms on one side of the body (opposite the half of the brain in which the seizure occurs). These are often referred to as "focal seizures."
- **Generalized onset seizure:** A seizure that starts from both halves of the brain. Generalized seizures lead to signs and symptoms on both sides of the body and are often referred to as "generalized seizures."
- **Unknown onset seizure:** A seizure with an unclear starting location in the brain. The seizure is either focal onset or generalized onset, but the exact onset zone cannot be determined. Seizures classified as unknown may be later classified as focal onset or generalized onset if more testing identifies the onset zone.

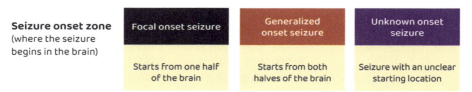

Figure 2.3.1 Seizure classification based on seizure onset zone.

The seizure onset zone may be determined by the signs and symptoms that appear at the onset of the seizure or by EEG. However, the onset of a seizure is not always witnessed, and some seizures that may appear to be generalized at first may actually be focal upon further evaluation.

Second classification: Level of awareness during a seizure

The second classification is based on the level of awareness during a seizure. The level of awareness is the individual's state of consciousness during a seizure and includes their "knowledge of self or environment."[62] Individuals experiencing seizures may either be aware or have impaired awareness:

- **Aware:** The individual does not experience a loss of consciousness and is aware that a seizure is happening. They may even be able to carry on a conversation or complete a task during a seizure. They are also likely to recall the events during a seizure after it ends.
- **Impaired awareness:** The individual may appear confused, is not aware a seizure is occurring, may not be able to respond, or may experience a loss of consciousness. After the seizure ends, the individual will typically not be able to fully recall the event.

Focal onset seizures are either aware or impaired awareness seizures. However, *all generalized onset seizures are presumed to have impaired awareness*. Figure 2.3.2 depicts the level of awareness during a seizure.

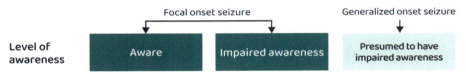

Figure 2.3.2 Level of awareness during a seizure.

Third classification: Motor or nonmotor

The third classification is based on the signs and symptoms of the seizure—what the seizure "looks" like, or how the individual feels or acts during the seizure. These are known as motor (movement) signs and nonmotor (without movement) signs and symptoms:

- **Motor signs** are uncontrolled physical movements experienced by the individual during the seizure that can be seen by others observing the individual.
- **Nonmotor signs and symptoms** are what the individual who is seizing experiences. These may be observed by others if they include a lack of movement, emotional outbursts, or a change in vital signs.

Motor signs and nonmotor signs and symptoms occur in both focal onset and generalized onset seizures.[62] Multiple signs and symptoms may occur within a seizure, often simultaneously.

Focal onset seizures are classified as motor *onset* or nonmotor *onset*, while generalized onset seizures are classified as motor or nonmotor (i.e., without the word "onset"). The difference is that focal seizures may start with motor signs and then change to include nonmotor signs and symptoms, or vice versa, while generalized onset seizures stay either as motor or nonmotor and do not usually change.

Focal onset seizures

Focal onset seizures are classified as motor onset or nonmotor onset, depending on what the *first* sign or symptom of the seizure is. The name of the seizure includes both the classification of the motor onset and the first sign that occurs. For example, if the first sign is uncontrolled physical movement, such as tonic movement, the focal onset seizure is classified as **motor onset** and termed a focal motor tonic seizure (or just focal tonic seizure). Focal onset seizures may be characterized by any of the following motor signs:

- **Automatisms:** Repetitive, often excessive actions involving the face, arms, or legs, performed without conscious thought or intention; may include lip-smacking, chewing, repetitive hand movements, or picking at the hair or clothing.[62,68,69]
- **Atonic events:** Sudden loss of muscle tone in the head, trunk, jaw, and limbs.[62] When these occur, the seizure is sometimes called a "drop seizure" because the individual may have a head drop or completely drop to the floor due to the sudden loss in muscle tone.[70]
- **Clonic movements:** Repetitive, rhythmic contractions or twitching (repeated stiffening and relaxing or jerking) of specific muscle groups of the limbs, face, or trunk.[71]
- **Epileptic spasms:** Sudden movements that last for one to two seconds and involve muscle contraction causing flexion (bending), extension (straightening), or mixed flexion-extension of a limb.[62]
- **Hyperkinetic movements:** Excessive, abnormal, and large involuntary movements that may include motions such as thrashing or leg pedaling.[12,62]
- **Myoclonic movements:** Sudden single or multiple involuntary muscle contractions that last less than a second.[62]
- **Tonic movements:** Sustained muscle contractions resulting in a sudden stiffness or tense posture, typically seen as an extension of the

limb.[62] Tonic movements may involve more than one limb and are typically short, lasting less than 20 seconds.[72]

If the *first* indication a seizure is occurring is something other than physical movement, the focal onset seizure is classified as **nonmotor onset** and may be characterized by any of the following nonmotor signs and symptoms:

- **Aura:** A sensation or symptom experienced at the onset of a neurological event.[73] Auras may start before or at the beginning of a seizure, and are sometimes known as a seizure warning signal. Auras are often the first noticeable symptom of a seizure, before any physical signs.[61] Auras may include sudden intense feelings of fear or joy, a feeling of déjà vu, numbness or tingling, unusual tastes or smells, visual disturbances, feeling dizzy, headaches, or nausea.[74]
- **Autonomic actions:** Actions that are controlled by the autonomic nervous system* that may include heart racing, feelings of hot or cold, goosebumps, drooling, or other symptoms such as gastrointestinal sensations.[67,68,75]
- **Behavioral arrest:** The abrupt stopping of talking or moving and the appearance of "freezing up."[69]
- **Cognitive symptoms:** Feelings of being confused and forgetting events around the time of the seizure.
- **Emotional symptoms:** Unexpected crying, screaming, laughing, or intense feelings of fear or anxiety.[69]
- **Sensory phenomena:** A feeling of detachment from self, intrusive thoughts, or an overall feeling of spinning or out-of-body experiences.[62] Sensory phenomena may include any of the senses and may present as flashing lights or spots of color or darkness; buzzing, drumming, ringing, and whistling sounds; tingling, numbness, pain, or shock-like sensations; a sense of movement; odors of burning, sulfur, alcohol, gas, garbage, barbecue, flowers; and bitter, salty, metallic, and sour taste.[62] **Somatosensory** symptoms may also occur; these are specific types of sensory phenomena that produce sensations related to touch, temperature, body position, and pain.[76]

---

* The autonomic nervous system regulates involuntary processes in the human body, including heart rate, digestion, and breathing.

Figure 2.3.3 summarizes focal onset seizures (motor onset and nonmotor onset) that may present with signs and symptoms described above.

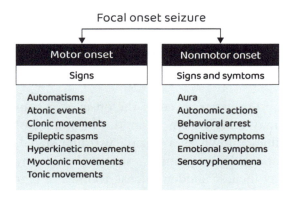

Figure 2.3.3 Focal onset seizure (motor onset or nonmotor onset).

Generalized onset seizures

Generalized onset seizures are all presumed impaired awareness seizures. Due to the impaired awareness that accompanies generalized onset seizures, *most* generalized onset seizures are classified as motor seizures since the individual experiencing the seizure is not able to recall any nonmotor signs and symptoms. A specific type of nonmotor generalized onset seizure is known as an absence seizure, described below.

A generalized onset seizure with uncontrolled physical movement is classified as a **motor** seizure. The naming of the seizure includes both the classification as a motor seizure and the specific motor signs that occur. A generalized onset seizure often involves multiple motor signs occurring in succession (i.e., one movement ends and is immediately followed by another). For example, if the seizure involves uncontrolled physical movement, such as tonic movement immediately followed by clonic movement, the generalized onset seizure is classified as **motor** and termed a generalized motor tonic-clonic seizure (or just generalized tonic-clonic seizure). Generalized onset seizures may be characterized by any of the following motor signs:

- **Atonic event:** Sudden loss of muscle tone in the head, trunk, jaw, and limbs.[62] When this occurs, the seizure is sometimes called a

"drop seizure" because the individual may have a head drop or completely drop to the floor due to the sudden loss in muscle tone.[70]
- **Clonic movements:** Repetitive, rhythmic contractions or twitching (repeated stiffening and relaxing or jerking) of specific muscle groups of the limbs, face, or trunk.[71]
- **Epileptic spasms:** Sudden movements that last for one to two seconds and involve muscle contraction causing flexion (bending), extension (straightening), or mixed flexion-extension of a limb.[62]
- **Myoclonic movements:** Sudden single or multiple involuntary muscle contractions that last less than a second.[62]
- **Myoclonic-atonic movements:** Myoclonic movements followed in succession by an atonic event.
- **Myoclonic-tonic-clonic movements:** Myoclonic movements followed by tonic-clonic movements.
- **Tonic movements:** Sustained muscle contractions resulting in a sudden stiffness or tense posture, typically seen as an extension of the limb.[62] Tonic movements may involve more than one limb and are typically short, lasting less than 20 seconds.[72]
- **Tonic-clonic movements:** Tonic movements in which the individual loses consciousness and the muscles suddenly contract (lasting about 10 to 20 seconds) followed immediately by clonic movements in which the muscles repetitively and rhythmically contract (lasting one or two minutes, or less).

A generalized onset seizure that is a nonmotor seizure is known as an **absence** seizure. In absence seizures, the individual may *appear* to be aware and awake and will stare blankly and not respond, as if daydreaming or not paying attention. However, these seizures are classified as impaired awareness and the individual typically has no memory of the event after it ends. Absence seizures are always generalized onset seizures and may be further classified as follows:

- **Typical absence seizure:** Activity suddenly stops, staring may last 10 to 20 seconds, and the individual may be confused for a few seconds after the event.[70]
- **Atypical absence seizure:** Seizure activity lasts longer than a typical absence seizure, approximately 20 seconds or longer, and is accompanied by motor signs such as a change in muscle tone, blinking or eyelid fluttering, lip-smacking, or hand motions.[70]

- **Myoclonic absence seizure:** Myoclonic movements associated with absence or a subtle impaired awareness.[77]
- **Eyelid myoclonia absence seizure:** Myoclonic jerks of the eyelids, along with brief periods of absence (typically lasting less than six seconds).[78]

Figure 2.3.4 summarizes generalized onset seizures (motor or nonmotor).

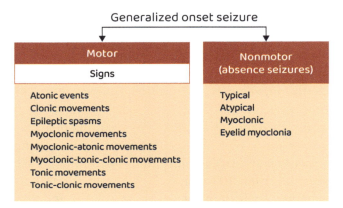

Figure 2.3.4 Generalized onset seizure (motor or nonmotor).

Unknown onset seizures

Unknown onset seizures are seizures with an unclear starting point in the brain. They may be classified as motor or nonmotor based on the signs and symptoms, or they may be unclassified if there is inadequate information.

Figure 2.3.5 summarizes unknown onset seizures.

Unknown onset seizure

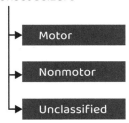

Figure 2.3.5 Unknown onset seizure.

Seizures do not always stay within the onset zone they start in. A seizure that begins as a focal onset seizure may spread to become a generalized seizure, termed "focal to bilateral seizure." One example is a focal to bilateral tonic-clonic seizure: the name of this seizure describes the initial onset zone (focal), includes the spread to both halves of the brain ("bilateral" means two-sided), and refers to the motor signs that occur (tonic-clonic).[79]

Figure 2.3.6 (on the next page) summarizes the full classification of seizures.

Observing a seizure and noting the level of awareness (aware versus impaired awareness), the signs and symptoms (motor versus nonmotor), and how long each last, along with the body parts involved (both arms or legs, just one side of the body, or the face) helps to classify it. Using a stopwatch (e.g., on a phone) helps determine the length of the signs and symptoms, and video recording the event may help identify the seizure onset zone. However, those observing an individual having a seizure should focus on ensuring the individual's safety and providing care as needed before attempting to video record it.

Nonmotor symptoms may be difficult to notice, as they are being experienced only by the individual having the seizure. When possible, the individual experiencing nonmotor symptoms should be encouraged to document what they are experiencing, along with the length of time the symptoms last.

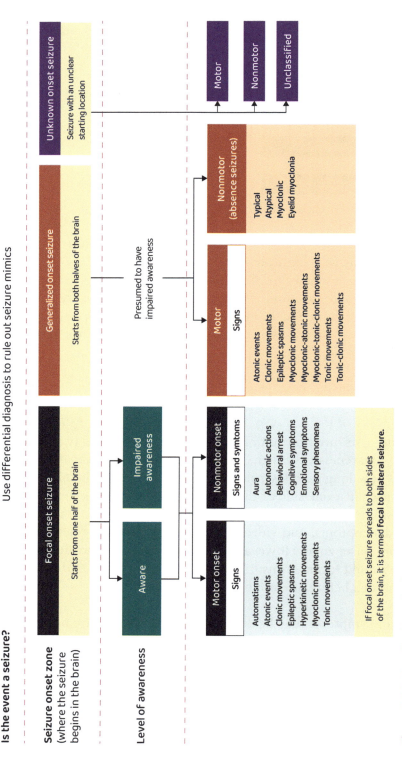

Figure 2.3.6 Classification of seizures.

2.4

Phases of a seizure

A river cuts through rock, not because of its power, but because of its persistence.
Jim Watkins

A seizure is often described in "phases." These phases include events happening right before, during, and after the seizure. The duration of the phases is variable, and individuals may move through them quickly, or the return to baseline may take a long time. Just as seizures can look different, so can each of the seizure phases.

Figure 2.4.1 depicts the phases of a seizure, with baseline before and after. The following explains the terms used:

- **Baseline:** This describes the typical feelings and activities of an individual when they are not experiencing a seizure; an individual will be at baseline before and after the phases of a seizure.
- **Preictal phase:** "Pre" means before; "ictal" means seizure. This stage typically happens seconds to minutes before the seizure begins and often includes symptoms that indicate a seizure will occur. The individual may notice an aura during the preictal phase.

- **Ictal phase:** This is the active phase of a seizure, which may include loss of consciousness, motor signs, or nonmotor signs and symptoms. This is usually the most obvious phase to the observer and is what is typically described as the actual seizure.
- **Postictal phase:** "Post" means after. This phase is after the seizure stops. The individual may experience impaired awareness during this phase, particularly following generalized tonic-clonic seizures, but this often resolves within minutes.[80] Headache, fatigue, weakness, motor impairments, and issues with cognition (such as memory impairments or confusion) may last for hours following a seizure, and some psychiatric and behavioral symptoms may last for days or weeks.[80] An example of a postictal condition with motor impairment is Todd's paralysis (also termed "paresis"), which is temporary paralysis in one or both sides of the body that may occur following focal onset seizures or focal to bilateral tonic-clonic seizures. It resolves within minutes to hours following a seizure.[62]

It is important to note that, because of the lasting effects of seizures, individuals should not do anything potentially dangerous during the postictal phase (e.g., drive a vehicle, play sports) until they return to baseline.

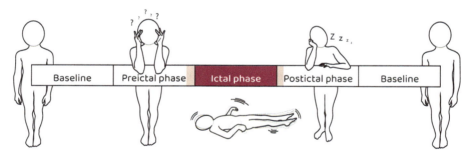

Figure 2.4.1 Phases of a seizure. In this figure, the ictal phase as shown applies to a generalized tonic-clonic seizure.

2.5 Classification of epilepsy

> Learn from yesterday, live for today, hope for tomorrow.
> The important thing is not to stop questioning.
> **Albert Einstein**

Differential diagnosis is used after an event to clarify if the event was a seizure mimic or a seizure (section 1.4). Further determination is made to decide if it is a provoked or an unprovoked seizure (section 2.2), and then to classify the seizure type (section 2.3). This section addresses the classification of epilepsy. Classification, or dividing into groups, is useful because it provides information about the nature of the condition, its severity, and the expected response to treatment. Antiseizure medications often target specific types of seizures and epilepsy, and some non-pharmaceutical treatments are very effective with certain types of epilepsy. Classification allows for predicting the development of comorbidities and prognosis, both short- and long-term. Classification also allows individuals with epilepsy and parents of children with epilepsy to connect with others who have similar types. Finally, classification helps with research. The current medical standard for classifying epilepsy as developed by the ILAE is shown in Figure 2.5.1. It includes classification on the basis of:

- Epilepsy types
- Etiology (cause)
- Epilepsy syndromes

As well, at each classification level, comorbidities are considered. The classification of epilepsy is important because the management of each classification may vary.

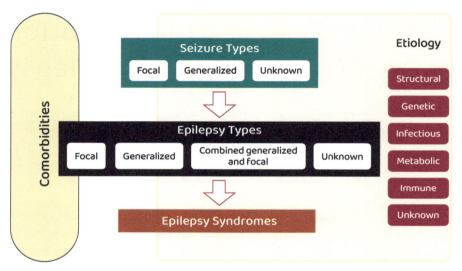

Figure 2.5.1 ILAE framework for classifying epilepsy. Adapted from *Epilepsia*, a journal of the ILAE. Used under a Creative Commons Attribution-Sharealike 4.0 International License https://creativecommons.org/licenses/by-sa/4.0/

Epilepsy types

As with seizure types, different epilepsy types are classified. Epilepsy type is based on the *main* type of seizure experienced, even though individuals with epilepsy may experience multiple types of seizures. The four epilepsy types are:

- **Focal epilepsy (also called focal onset epilepsy)**, which is characterized by focal onset seizures and is the most common type of epilepsy in both children and adults.[81] In children, focal epilepsy comprises about two-thirds of all cases of epilepsy.[81]

- **Generalized epilepsy** (also called **generalized onset epilepsy**), which is characterized by generalized onset seizures. It is less common than focal epilepsy and usually starts in childhood.
- **Combined generalized and focal epilepsy** (also called **combined generalized and focal onset epilepsy**), which is characterized by both focal onset and generalized onset seizures.
- **Unknown epilepsy** (also called **unknown onset epilepsy**), which cannot be clearly distinguished as focal, generalized, or combined generalized and focal. Unknown epilepsy may later be reevaluated and reclassified into a specific epilepsy type, once more information is obtained.

Etiology (cause)

Etiology is the cause of a condition. The causes of epilepsy are the same as the causes of unprovoked seizures; they may be:

- **Structural:** There is a distinct abnormality of the brain.
- **Genetic:** The cause is closely associated with pathologic changes in one or more genes.
- **Infectious:** The individual had a previous (not acute) infection in the brain.
- **Metabolic:** The individual has a metabolic disorder.
- **Immune:** There has been an alteration in the body's defense system against infections.
- **Unknown:** There is no definitive cause.

Causes of epilepsy are addressed in Chapter 6.

Epilepsy syndromes

An epilepsy syndrome is a group of symptoms consistently occurring together, associated with the diagnosis of epilepsy. A more formal definition is "a characteristic cluster of clinical and EEG features, often supported by etiologic findings (structural, genetic, metabolic, immune, and infectious)."[7] Epilepsy syndromes are classified by age of onset, and many begin in infancy or childhood. When epilepsy syndromes begin at a predictable age, they are referred to as "age dependent." Epilepsy syndromes may resolve on their own, or they may evolve into other types of epilepsy or another epilepsy syndrome as the individual ages.

Epilepsy syndromes are addressed in Chapter 7.

Comorbidities

Comorbidities are conditions that coexist with another condition in an individual.

Comorbidities often occur with epilepsy: about half of all people with epilepsy will have at least one comorbidity, and roughly 70 percent of children with epilepsy have at least one comorbidity.[21] Comorbidities associated with epilepsy may impact any area of the body, and they may resolve if the epilepsy resolves or they may persist. For many individuals with epilepsy, comorbidities may be more challenging than the seizures themselves.[32,82]

Comorbidities are addressed in Chapter 9.

Note that the field of epilepsy is continually evolving, and the classification of seizures and epilepsy has changed over the years. You may find in the literature you read that some "old" terms are mixed in with some "new" ones. This book uses the most up-to-date terms at the time of writing.[83] Appendix 3 (online) includes seizure and epilepsy terminology.

Emma continued to have seizures every few days in the beginning, so her diagnosis of epilepsy was made quite early. We tried a lot of different antiseizure medications: some worked well, and others had unpleasant side effects and we had to stop them.

Despite our roller-coaster ride with the medications, we were finally able to be discharged and go home and join her brother, Jake, and try to put our life together. We left the hospital feeling a bit anxious as we knew it was likely a matter of time before she had another seizure. I worried if she would have a seizure and I would sleep through it, or where we would be when it happened.

Just a few days after bringing her home, while she was napping, I watched her sweet face start to make some funny expressions, with her nose twitching back and forth and her eyes, although still closed, squinting on and off. I first thought perhaps she was dreaming. It took me a few minutes to realize this was probably a seizure. This was still all so new to me, and I quickly learned that no two seizures look the same, even in the same person.

2.6 Overview of epilepsy management

> The human spirit is stronger than anything that can happen to it.
> **George C. Scott**

Epilepsy management is complex. Epilepsy may evolve over time as the individual gets older, so the evaluation of the condition and its management is ongoing. Clinical expertise can vary, so it is important to know that information about management in this book may be different from practice among hospitals and treatment centers. Furthermore, management is not "one size fits all"; it must be customized. Epilepsy management in this section is addressed under the following headings:

- Important terminology
- Why manage epilepsy?
- How is epilepsy managed?
- Evidence-based medicine, shared decision-making, and family- and person-centered care

Important terminology

One of the main goals of epilepsy management is to *prevent, reduce,* or *stop* seizures. Some related important terms to understand include:

- **Seizure control:** Effective epilepsy management that results in a decrease in frequency, severity, and/or duration of seizures.
- **Seizure freedom:** A set period without any seizures; the ultimate goal of epilepsy management.
- **Remission:** A state where an individual with epilepsy is seizure-free for at least six months. Remission criteria vary, however, and for some individuals, a longer time period may be used (such as two years or five years).
- **Resolved:** A state where an individual with epilepsy has remained seizure-free for the last 10 years, with no antiseizure medications for the last 5 years, or the individual had an age-dependent epilepsy syndrome and is past the applicable age for this diagnosis (i.e., self-limited neonatal or infantile epilepsy syndromes).[5]

Why manage epilepsy?

Management of epilepsy is important for the following reasons:

- **To protect the brain from damage:** Epileptic seizures may lead to damage of areas in the brain, especially when they are prolonged or uncontrolled.
- **To protect organs and body systems from damage:** Epileptic seizures (especially those with motor signs) may lead to injuries and lesions in various body organs (e.g., kidneys or liver), or body systems (e.g., cardiovascular or musculoskeletal systems).
- **To prevent status epilepticus:** This condition, in which seizures last more than five minutes or occur in close succession (one after the other, without a return to baseline), is life-threatening.[2]
- **To prevent SUDEP (sudden unexpected death in epilepsy):** This rare complication of epilepsy is named to describe the unexpected death of an individual with epilepsy when no other cause of death can be found.

- **To ensure safety and prevent injury:** Individuals with epilepsy are at an increased risk of accidental injuries from falls, motor vehicle accidents, and accidents around water, fire, and in other activities.
- **To improve quality of life:** Seizure control correlates with the ability to participate fully in life, including social activities, physical activities, education, employment, driving, and independent living.

How is epilepsy managed?

The management of epilepsy generally includes:

- **Pharmaceutical treatments,** involving the use of antiseizure medications, either as monotherapy or polytherapy
- **Non-pharmaceutical treatments,** involving the ketogenic diet, neuromodulation (repetitive electrical discharges administered through a device), and epilepsy surgery
- **Other medications or supplements,** including vitamins or medical cannabis

Pharmaceutical treatments are generally tried first. However, some epilepsy syndromes and drug-resistant epilepsy (when two appropriately used antiseizure medications fail to achieve seizure freedom) are best managed with non-pharmaceutical treatments or other medications or supplements. Pharmaceutical treatments, non-pharmaceutical treatments, and other medications or supplements can be used with the same individual and at the same time.

Management options for epilepsy are shown in Table 2.6.1. Epilepsy management is addressed in detail in Chapter 8.

Table 2.6.1 Management options for epilepsy

MANAGEMENT	DESCRIPTION	INDICATIONS FOR USE
Pharmaceutical treatments		
Monotherapy	One antiseizure medication (may try a different medication if the first doesn't work)	All types of epilepsy, generally tried first
Polytherapy	More than one antiseizure medication given at the same time (may try different combinations)	All types of epilepsy, when monotherapy does not work
Non-pharmaceutical treatments		
Ketogenic diet	Specialized diet with a very low amount of carbohydrates	Used when polytherapy does not work, or when the epilepsy type, epilepsy cause, or epilepsy syndrome is more responsive to non-pharmaceutical management
Neuromodulation	Repetitive electrical discharges administered through a device (for the management of epilepsy, these devices are surgically implanted)	
Epilepsy surgery	Surgery to areas of the brain where seizures are thought to start or spread to	
Other medications and supplements		
Medications	Medications other than antiseizure medication include: • Immunotherapies (treatments that alter the immune system) • Steroids (medications with anti-inflammatory properties) • ACTH (a type of hormone therapy)	Used when the epilepsy type, epilepsy cause, or epilepsy syndrome is known to be responsive to a particular medication
Vitamins	Dietary supplements	Used in epilepsy syndromes known to be responsive to a particular vitamin
Medical cannabis	A pharmaceutical form of the cannabis plant	Used in epilepsy types and epilepsy syndromes known to be responsive to cannabis

Evidence-based medicine, shared decision-making, and family- and person-centered care

When a child is diagnosed with epilepsy, the whole family is affected: parents, siblings, and extended family members. Family-centered care is a way of ensuring that care is planned around the whole family, not just the child with the condition.*[84] It can be thought of as a meeting of experts who pool their knowledge to jointly develop the most appropriate plan of care for the child. The parent is the expert on their child, while the professional is the expert on the condition and its treatment. Professionals who practice family-centered care see themselves not as the sole authority but as a partner with the parent in the provision of care for the child. Family-centered care and person-centered care are closely related. The latter evolves from the former as the child grows. In person-centered care, insofar as cognitive capacity allows, the individual is an active participant and decision-maker in their own medical care. The change from family-centered care to person-centered care is gradual, and parents and medical professionals can help facilitate the shift over time.

Evidence-based medicine (or evidence-based practice) is "the conscientious, explicit, and judicious use of current best evidence in making decisions about the care of individual patients."[85] It combines the best available external clinical evidence from research with the clinical expertise of the professional.[85] Family priorities and preferences are also considered.[86]

Best practice in managing epilepsy is having a multidisciplinary team skilled in providing medical care and engaging with the family in a shared decision-making model, a process in which the family is actively involved in making decisions about medical treatment and care. The key to shared decision-making is incorporating the principles of evidence-based medicine.[87]

---

* Family-centered care is also termed "family-centered service." CanChild, a Canadian research centre, defines the term as care that is "made up of a set of values, attitudes, and approaches to services for children with special needs and their families. [It] recognizes that **each family is unique**; that the family is the **constant in the child's life**; and that they are the **experts on the child's abilities and needs**. The family works with service providers to make informed decisions about the services and supports the child and family receive."

2.7

Sudden unexpected death in epilepsy

> Start where you are.
> Use what you have.
> Do what you can.
>
> **Arthur Ashe**

As noted in section 2.6, preventing sudden unexpected death in epilepsy (SUDEP) is one of the important reasons for managing epilepsy. SUDEP is the unexpected death of an individual with epilepsy when no other cause of death can be found. SUDEP occurs in about 1 in 1,000 individuals with epilepsy each year.[88] Children and adults are affected at a similar rate.[89]

The cause of SUDEP is unknown, though suspected causes include an irregular heart rhythm or breathing difficulties following a seizure, though SUDEP may also occur without any evidence of a seizure. The risk of SUDEP increases with:[88–90]

- Poor seizure control
- Generalized tonic-clonic seizures (particularly when they occur in unattended individuals at night)

- Drug-resistant epilepsy
- Missed antiseizure medication doses
- Alcohol consumption

SUDEP frequently occurs at night or during sleep, and although nighttime supervision or monitoring may help prevent it,[21] the best way to decrease the risk of SUDEP is to optimize seizure control through effective epilepsy management.

Key points Chapter 2

- Classification of seizures and epilepsy is important because it provides information about the nature of the condition, its severity, and expected response to treatment.
- Seizures are classified into provoked or unprovoked, and the causes of each vary. Provoked seizures are not typically associated with epilepsy; unprovoked seizures are more often associated with epilepsy.
- Seizures are classified based on where the seizure begins in the brain (seizure onset zone); focal onset seizures start from one half of the brain and generalized onset seizures start from both halves of the brain. If the starting point of the seizure in the brain is unclear, the seizure is classified as unknown onset.
- Seizures are classified based on the level of awareness during a seizure. Focal onset seizures are either aware or impaired awareness seizures. However, all generalized onset seizures are presumed to have impaired awareness.
- Seizures are classified based on the signs and symptoms of the seizure—what the seizure "looks" like, or how the individual feels or acts during the seizure.
- Motor signs include uncontrolled physical movement, and non-motor signs and symptoms include auras, feelings, emotions, and sensory phenomena.
- Seizures occur in phases that include events that happen immediately before the start of a seizure (preictal phase), during the seizure (ictal phase), and immediately after the seizure (postictal phase).
- Epilepsy is classified based on the type, cause, and syndrome, and classification includes consideration for comorbidities.
- One of the main goals in epilepsy management is to prevent, reduce, or stop seizures. Epilepsy management is important to protect the brain and organ systems from damage, ensure safety and prevent injury, and improve quality of life for individuals with epilepsy.
- Epilepsy management is complex and may involve the use of pharmaceuticals such as antiseizure medications, non-pharmaceutical options including the ketogenic diet, neuromodulation, epilepsy surgery, or other medications and supplements, including vitamins or medical cannabis. Pharmaceutical, non-pharmaceutical, and

other medications or supplements can be used with the same individual and at the same time.
- The best practice of managing epilepsy is having a multidisciplinary team skilled in providing medical care and engaging with the family in a shared decision-making model.
- Sudden unexpected death in epilepsy (SUDEP) is the unexpected death of an individual with epilepsy when no other cause of death can be found. The best way to decrease the risk of SUDEP is to optimize seizure control through effective epilepsy management.

Chapter 3

The nervous system

Section 3.1 Introduction 59
Section 3.2 The brain 61
Section 3.3 Neurons 70
Section 3.4 Seizure threshold 73
Key points Chapter 3 75

3.1 Introduction

> Biology gives you a brain. Life turns it into a mind.
> **Jeffrey Eugenides**

Understanding the nervous system is important in understanding seizures and epilepsy. The central nervous system (CNS) is composed of the brain and spinal cord. The nerves are part of the peripheral nervous system. Nerves carry signals from the brain and spinal cord to the body and from the body back to the brain and spinal cord. See Figure 3.1.1.

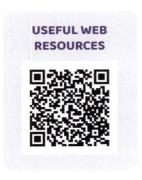

USEFUL WEB RESOURCES

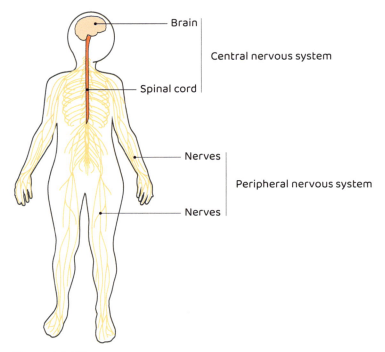

Figure 3.1.1 The nervous system.

3.2 The brain

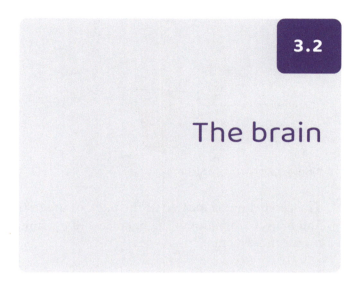

If the human brain were so simple that we could understand it, we would be so simple that we couldn't.

George Edgin Pugh

Parts of the brain

The brain is divided into several distinct parts that serve important functions. See Figure 3.2.1.

The **cerebrum** is the front and upper part of the brain; it is also the largest part of the brain. The outer layer of the cerebrum is known as the **cerebral cortex** (see Figure 3.2.2). The cerebral cortex has a large surface area and, due to its folds, appears wrinkled. Different regions of the cerebral cortex have different functions. The cerebral cortex is responsible for the majority of voluntary actions, as well as thinking, learning, consciousness, personality and many of the senses.[91]

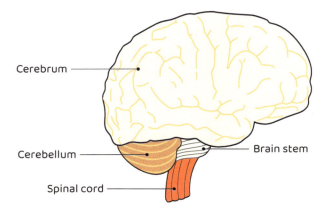

Figure 3.2.1 Parts of the brain.

The **cerebellum** is located at the back of the brain, under the cerebrum, and helps with maintaining balance and posture, coordination, and fine motor movements.[92]

The **brain stem** is the bottom part of the brain that connects the cerebrum to the **spinal cord**. It also serves as a relay station for messages between different parts of the body and the cerebral cortex. Many functions responsible for survival are located here (e.g., breathing and heart rate).

The cerebrum is divided into two halves, referred to as hemispheres (see Figure 3.2.2). In general, the right hemisphere controls the left side of the body; the left hemisphere controls the right side of the body. Therefore, damage or seizure activity on the right half of the cerebrum will impact the left side of the body and vice versa. Communication between the two halves occurs in the **corpus callosum,** located in the center of the cerebrum.

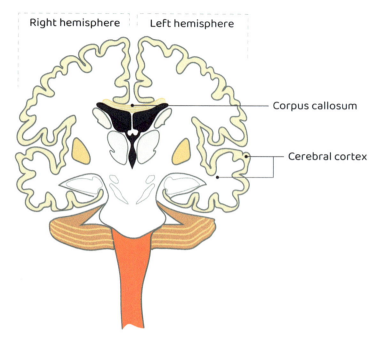

Figure 3.2.2 Vertical cross-section of the brain.

Cerebral cortex

The cerebral cortex is divided into four lobes: frontal, parietal, temporal, and occipital (see Figure 3.2.3).

Each lobe is responsible for different functions in the body. Seizures with onset zones in each lobe produce distinct signs and symptoms, which can help to localize seizure onset. However, relying on signs and symptoms alone to localize seizure onset must be done carefully because some seizures might start in deep brain regions and spread to other brain areas. In addition, if there has been an earlier brain injury or abnormal brain development in an individual, some functions typically associated with one area of the brain might be relocated to different areas.

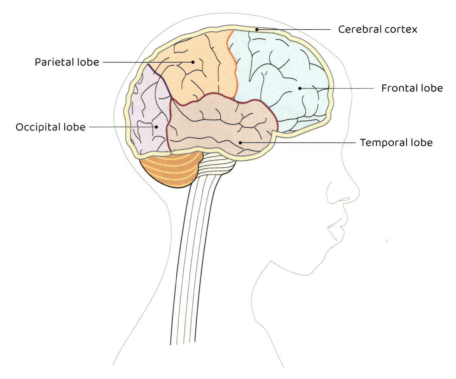

Figure 3.2.3 Lobes of the cerebral cortex.

Typical seizure signs and symptoms associated with each cerebral cortex lobe are presented in Table 3.2.1.

Table 3.2.1 Typical seizure signs and symptoms associated with lobes of the cerebral cortex

CEREBRAL CORTEX LOBE	FUNCTION	TYPICAL SEIZURE SIGNS AND SYMPTOMS
Frontal lobe	Responsible for personality, thinking, emotions, decision-making, judgment, self-control, attention, memory, and speech.[91,93] Responsible for voluntary muscle control and movement along the motor cortex.	Brief seizures (often less than 30 seconds) occur multiple times per day and include vocalization (producing sound).[94] These seizures often occur from sleep and can include tonic movements, clonic movements, and complex motor movements such as cycling or rocking and other types of hyperkinetic movements.[94,95]
Parietal lobe	Controls the understanding of spatial relationships, identification of objects, interpretation of pain and touch, and the spoken language.[91,93] Receives sensory information along the somatosensory cortex.	Somatosensory symptoms are common and include auras, body distortion, visual hallucinations, and sensations such as numbness and tingling, or dizziness.[94,95] Seizures beginning in the parietal lobe often spread to other lobes.[94]
Temporal lobe	Involved in short-term memory, speech, musical rhythm, emotion, and some degree of smell recognition.[91,93]	Seizures in this lobe are typically longer (2 to 3 minutes) compared to seizures in the frontal lobe and include auras and confusion after the seizure ends.[95] These seizures may include behavioral arrest, automatisms, and varying levels of impaired awareness.[94] Taste and smell symptoms may also occur.[95]
Occipital lobe	Vision.[93]	These seizures may include visual aura, eye blinking, or crossed eyes.[95]

Motor cortex and somatosensory cortex

Within the frontal lobes (on both halves of the brain) is the motor cortex, which is responsible for voluntary movements. Within the parietal lobes (on both halves of the brain) is the somatosensory cortex, which is responsible for receiving sensory information.

Figure 3.2.4 shows the right motor cortex (in teal) and the left somatosensory cortex (in orange). The teal and orange arrows depict the fact that each cortex, in general, controls the opposite side of the body (i.e., the left motor cortex controls the right side of the body and vice versa; the left somatosensory cortex receives information from the right side of the body and vice versa). Note that each point along each cortex corresponds to a specific area of the body. The motor cortex and the somatosensory cortex are replicated on both sides of the brain, but only one of each is shown in Figure 3.2.4.

Movements in the body are coordinated by communication between the motor and somatosensory cortices: when part of the body is moved, the motor cortex generates the movement, and the somatosensory cortex receives information about the movement and loops it back to the motor cortex. This communication loop allows for smooth, coordinated movements. Disruption in this communication loop due to seizures results in the motor signs and nonmotor signs and symptoms associated with seizures.

The motor signs or somatosensory (nonmotor) signs and symptoms during a seizure are a product of where in the motor or somatosensory cortices the seizure occurs. Making note of the body areas affected during a seizure can help with identifying the seizure onset zone.

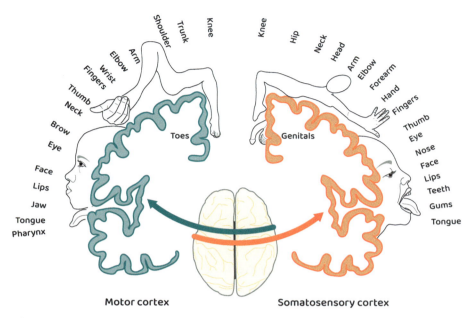

Figure 3.2.4 Motor cortex and somatosensory cortex. Adapted from Sensory Homunculus Illustration, Anatomy & Physiology, Connexions website (2013). Used under Creative Commons Attribution 3.0 Unported License https://creativecommons.org/licenses/by/3.0/deed.en

Other areas of the brain

Several other areas of the brain that control speech, memory, and learning are important in understanding seizures and epilepsy. These include Broca's area, Wernicke's area, the hippocampus, and the amygdala.

a) Broca's area and Wernicke's area

Typically, the dominant half of the brain is the one opposite to the dominant hand, with few exceptions.[96,97] Broca's area and Wernicke's area, shown in Figure 3.2.5, are usually found in the dominant half of the brain.

Broca's area is in the dominant frontal lobe and Wernicke's area is in the dominant temporal lobe. Seizures in these two areas lead to "aphasia," which means difficulty with putting thoughts into words, or difficulty understanding verbal language.[97,98]

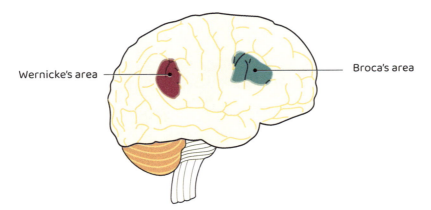

Figure 3.2.5 Broca's area and Wernicke's area.

b) Hippocampus and amygdala

Unlike Broca's area and Wernicke's area, the hippocampus and amygdala are paired, meaning these structures are found in both halves of the brain and lie deep within the temporal lobe in an area known as the medial temporal lobe (see Figure 3.2.6).

- **The hippocampus** is primarily associated with memory, particularly long-term memory storage and consolidation, and decision-making.[99] An example of the hippocampus being involved in seizures is a condition known as hippocampal sclerosis. In this condition, the hippocampus hardens and shrinks, and the individual experiences intellectual issues such as memory loss and behavioral changes.[100,101] Individuals with hippocampal sclerosis frequently experience seizures in the temporal lobe, and the seizures are often drug resistant.[101]
- **The amygdala** is a small almond-shaped structure at the end of the hippocampus responsible for emotional processes, including processing memories and regulating emotions and behaviors (both positive and negative).[102] Individuals with frequent temporal lobe seizures may experience damage to the amygdala leading to emotional and behavioral issues including depression, irritability, and confusion.[103]

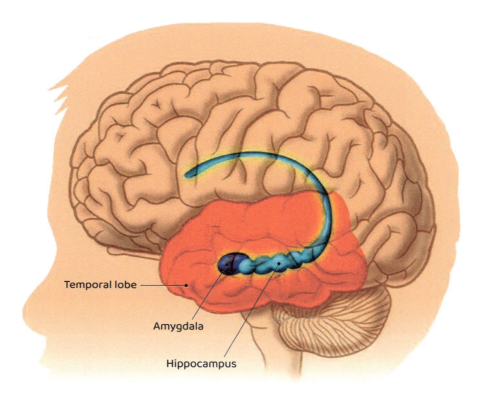

Figure 3.2.6 Hippocampus and amygdala within the medial temporal lobe. Reproduced with kind permission from BrainHQ.

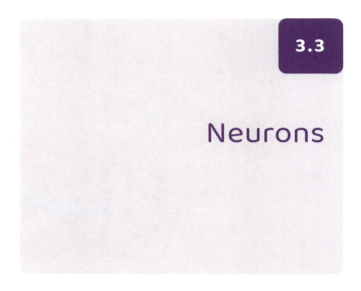

3.3 Neurons

> You can do what you decide to do—but you cannot decide what you will decide to do.
>
> **Sam Harris**

Neurons are the smallest unit of the nervous system, and there are billions of them in the brain and spinal cord. They are electrically excitable cells and carry information (signals) between the CNS and the rest of the body as electrical impulses through a web-like structure from neuron to neuron, or from neurons to other cells in the body.[104]

There are three common types of neurons:

- **Motor neurons,** which carry information *from* the CNS *to* a muscle
- **Sensory neurons,** which carry information *from* the rest of the body *to* the CNS
- **Interneurons** (also known as "relay neurons"), which carry information *between* neurons

Electrical activity moves through and out of a neuron to the next neuron or cell via a complex process. For a neuron to "fire" and send a signal, a critical electrical charge, called the "depolarization threshold," must be reached. The neuron consistently fires at full strength every time the threshold is reached, regardless of the strength of the stimulus. (This principle is known as "all or none.") If the threshold is not reached, no signal is sent. An analogy is a light switch: it's either fully on or off; there is no partial signal.

Once the depolarization threshold is reached, charged particles, called ions (such as sodium, potassium, and chloride), flow rapidly through channels in the neuron's membrane. This movement of ions creates the electrical impulse that travels along the neuron.

The junction between the sending neuron and the receiving neuron or cell is called a synapse, where special chemicals called neurotransmitters are released. These neurotransmitters carry the signal across the synapse by either stimulating (exciting) the next neuron or cell to take action or preventing (inhibiting) it from doing so.

Neurons and seizures

Recall that a seizure is uncontrolled, abnormal electrical activity of the brain. The neuron is the center of the abnormal electrical activity that leads to a seizure. Seizure activity, however, occurs in networks of multiple neurons, not just in single neurons (see Figure 3.3.1).

When neurons fire in atypical and uncontrolled ways, a seizure may occur. During a seizure, the ability of the neurons to regulate the signals is disrupted and the electrical activity that occurs is uncontrolled. However, not all uncontrolled electrical activity in neurons will lead to a seizure. For a seizure to occur, the seizure threshold must be reached (see section 3.4).

More information on neurons is included in Appendix 4 (online).

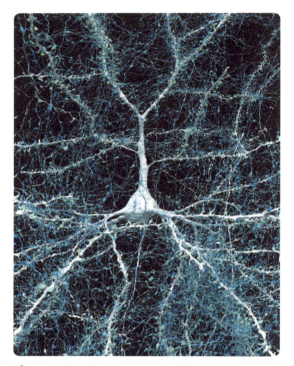

Figure 3.3.1 A single neuron (white) with thousands of connections to multiple other neurons. Reproduced with kind permission from Daniel Berger, Lichtman Lab, Harvard University.

3.4 Seizure threshold

> When there is no turning back,
> then we should concern ourselves only
> with the best way of going forward.
> **Paulo Coelho**

A seizure threshold is the theoretical sum of the various triggers that are likely enough for the abnormal electrical activity to initiate a seizure. Put another way, a seizure threshold is the point at which an individual's brain is likely to experience a seizure.

Note that seizure thresholds vary from person to person and throughout the lifetime.[2] A person with a low seizure threshold is more likely to experience a seizure, while someone with a high seizure threshold is less likely to experience a seizure, even under the same circumstances. This is why one person may experience a seizure, while another does not, even when both are faced with the same circumstances.

Seizure thresholds are important to understand in the management of epilepsy since many antiseizure medications increase the seizure threshold (e.g., by acting on neurotransmitters), making seizures less likely.

Currently, no specific formula or calculation exists to determine an individual's seizure threshold. Still, the theoretical seizure threshold is important because it is based on seizure risk factors, some of which may be altered to decrease the chances of having a seizure. In an individual already at risk for having seizures (based on history, a diagnosis of epilepsy, or other factors, described in Chapters 1 and 2), triggers that lower the seizure threshold (making seizures more likely) include:[105]

- Certain medications
- Dehydration
- Delaying or missing a dose of antiseizure medication
- Fever
- Flashing lights (in some epilepsy syndromes)
- Hyperventilation (in some epilepsy syndromes)
- Infections
- Malnutrition or fasting
- Menstrual cycle or other hormonal changes (in some cases)
- Illicit drug or alcohol use
- Sleep deprivation
- Trauma or injury

Key points Chapter 3

- The central nervous system comprises the brain and spinal cord. The nerves are part of the peripheral nervous system and communicate signals from the brain and spinal cord to the body and from the body back to the brain and spinal cord.
- The brain is divided into several distinct parts that serve important functions.
- The cerebral cortex (the outer layer of the cerebrum) has four lobes: frontal lobe, parietal lobe, temporal lobe, and occipital lobe. Seizures with onset in each lobe produce distinct signs and symptoms, which can help to localize seizure onset.
- The motor cortex and somatosensory cortex are specialized areas on the cerebral cortex. The motor signs or somatosensory symptoms during a seizure are a product of where in the motor or somatosensory cortex the seizure occurs.
- Broca's area and Wernicke's area are found in the frontal and temporal lobe and are responsible for language and speech.
- The hippocampus and amygdala are found deep in the temporal lobe in an area known as the medial temporal lobe and are responsible for memory, behavior, and emotions.
- Neurons are electrically excitable cells and carry information between the CNS and the rest of the body as electrical impulses.
- When neurons fire in atypical and uncontrolled ways, a seizure can occur.
- For a seizure to occur, the seizure threshold must be met. A seizure threshold is the point at which an individual's brain is likely to experience a seizure. A person with a low seizure threshold is more likely to experience a seizure, while someone with a high seizure threshold is less likely to experience a seizure, even in the same circumstances.
- Common triggers that lower the seizure threshold include sleep deprivation, fever, and infections.

Chapter 4

EEG and seizure detection

Section 4.1 Introduction to EEG 79
Section 4.2 What happens during EEG? 80
Section 4.3 Interpreting the EEG recording 86
Section 4.4 Phases of a seizure and EEG 92
Section 4.5 Seizure recording and detection 95
Key points Chapter 4 102

4.1

Introduction to EEG

You can't stop the waves, but you can learn how to surf.
Jon Kabat-Zinn

Electroencephalography, commonly known as EEG, measures and records the brain's electrical activity, generating a visual graph of brain waves. EEG allows medical professionals to interpret abnormal brain wave activity and specific EEG patterns that can indicate epilepsy. The main uses of EEG in epilepsy are to determine whether an individual is experiencing an epileptic seizure, to provide information to help evaluate the risk of recurrence of epileptic seizures, and to aid in diagnosing epilepsy.

USEFUL WEB RESOURCES

Video EEG (VEEG) involves the audiovisual recording of the individual while simultaneously measuring and recording brain wave activity. VEEG is considered the gold standard for diagnosing epilepsy.[41] The term EEG is used throughout this book, and it may or may not include the simultaneous audiovisual recording (i.e., VEEG).

4.2 What happens during EEG?

> The master key of knowledge is, indeed, a persistent and frequent questioning.
> **Peter Abelard**

During EEG, the medical professional evaluates the measured and recorded brain wave activity and observes the individual's level of awareness, motor signs, and nonmotor signs and symptoms. In addition, any unusual signs and symptoms can be indicated by the individual undergoing testing, or the parent of a child, by pushing an event button connected to the EEG system. If the individual starts to experience an aura, for example, they push the event button, and the medical professional examines the EEG recording at the time to determine if abnormal brain wave activity is present. A timed paper log or journal may also be used by the individual or parent to document events. This can be reviewed later and compared to the EEG recording.

EEG records only live events, however, so it is possible that no events will occur during EEG. If certain triggers are identified for the individual, those can be used to try to induce a seizure during EEG. Watching flashing lights, hyperventilating (breathing rapidly), closing eyes, opening eyes, and other actions are often performed during EEG to try and trigger an event.[106] Medical professionals may also request that the individual be sleep deprived since lack of sleep may be a trigger for seizures.[107] Some seizures occur more often with sleep, so an overnight stay in the hospital may help capture events related to sleep.

EEG can be done in either outpatient or inpatient settings. Typically, an outpatient EEG test lasts from 20 minutes to several hours, and an inpatient EEG test lasts from one to several days (or weeks in rare instances).

The process of EEG is depicted in Figure 4.2.1.

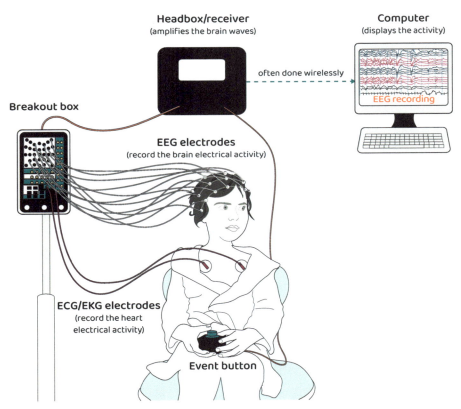

Figure 4.2.1 Process of EEG.

Electrode placement

During EEG, small metal discs known as electrodes are placed on the scalp (or inside the skull) that sense and record electrical activity in groups of neurons close to the electrode.[108] Trained technologists place the electrodes in specific areas on the scalp, which correlate to areas of the cerebral cortex. Typically, a small amount of gel is placed beneath the electrodes to help sense and record electrographic activity. The electrodes do *not* shock the individual.

The electrical activity sensed and recorded is known as "electrographic activity." The leads from the electrodes connect to a breakout box, which is connected to a headbox (receiver) to amplify the brain waves and allow visualization of the electrographic activity on a computer. What results is the EEG recording, used by medical professionals to interpret the brain's electrical activity.

Different types of electrodes may be used depending on factors such as the age of the individual and the expected length of the EEG test. These include:

- **Scalp electrodes:** These are placed directly onto the scalp and secured with paste or glue, and can be made of metal, gold plate, pure gold, or gelatinous materials. A child with scalp electrodes is shown in Figure 4.2.2.
- **Helmet or cap electrodes:** These are built into a helmet or cap, and the whole device is placed on the head. Though helmets or caps may appear easier to apply, individual electrodes, such as scalp electrodes, are often preferred because they typically result in better quality EEG recordings.
- **MRI-compatible electrodes:** These are used when MRI (magnetic resonance imaging) is needed while the electrodes are attached to the scalp.
- **Intracranial electrodes:** "Intra" means inside, and "cranial" refers to the skull. Intracranial electrodes are surgically placed inside the skull, inside the brain, or directly on the surface of the brain. These are used when a more detailed test is needed.

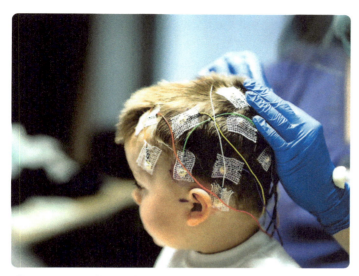

Figure 4.2.2 A child with scalp electrodes in place.

A commonly used pattern of electrode placement is known as the International 10–20 system (or simply, the 10–20 system). The 10 and the 20 indicate the percentage distance between electrodes. That is, the electrodes are placed at points that are either 10 or 20 percent of the total distance of bony landmarks on the skull, measured either front to back or left to right.[109] Figure 4.2.3 is a top view of a scalp (nose pointing up) with electrodes placed in a 10–20 system.

The 10–20 system is useful as it creates a standard for those placing the electrodes, and it allows for varying head shapes and sizes. Placing the electrodes can be a lengthy process as it involves taking measurements, followed by accurately placing many electrodes, typically between 21 and 30.

The numbered electrodes correspond to specific areas of the cerebral cortex; each is identified by letters and numbers. The letters represent lobes of the cerebral cortex and the numbers represent various areas on each hemisphere. Note that the midline uses letters only.[109]

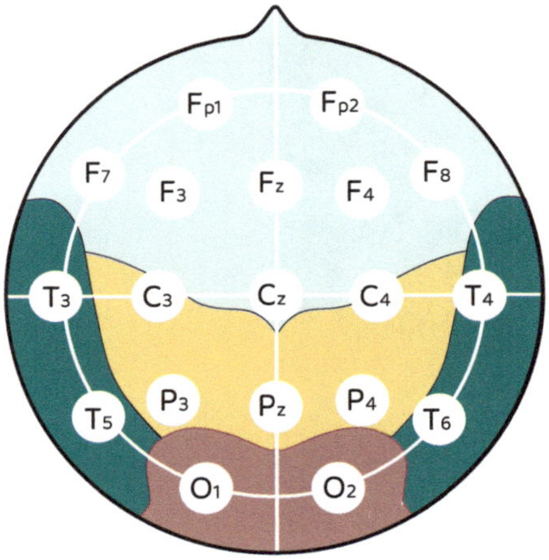

Figure 4.2.3 Placement of EEG electrodes using the International 10–20 system. Fp= frontopolar (in the frontal lobe), F= frontal, P= parietal, O= occipital, T= temporal. The left hemisphere is represented by odd numbers, the right hemisphere is represented by even numbers, and the midline is represented by "z"). Adapted with kind permission from Dr. Plass-Oude Bos.

By using a standard electrode placement system, the EEG recording can be organized into channels displayed on the computer. Channels are groups of two or more electrodes capturing activity that is reported as a single output. A common arrangement of channels organized by electrode pairs near to each other is called a "bipolar montage" ("bi" means two). In this way, the activity between two groups of neighboring neurons is combined, and orderly arrangements of channels are used to quickly compare areas of the brain to note atypical electrical activity, which may indicate seizures.

Figure 4.2.4 shows the EEG recording arranged in a bipolar montage, along with the electrode placement. The pairs of letters and numbers on the left side of the recording correspond to the electrode placement. Each pair of electrodes represents a channel (i.e., Fp1 and F7 form the first channel). The full list of channels (in this order) is a bipolar montage. In this example, the left hemisphere is displayed at the top half of the recording and the right hemisphere at the bottom half of the recording. The bipolar montage could also be displayed as alternating left and right hemispheres or by ordering from front to back. This comparison is useful in determining the location of the seizure onset zone.

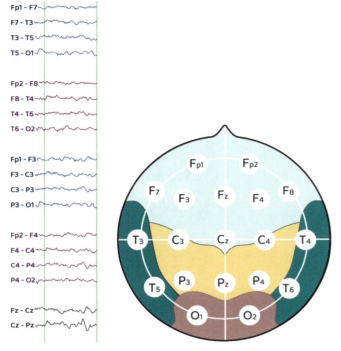

Figure 4.2.4 Bipolar montage using the International 10–20 system. Adapted with kind permission from Dr. Plass-Oude Bos.

ECGs and EMGs

In addition to EEG electrodes placed on the head, other electrodes may be placed elsewhere to record other electrical activity.

Electrodes are placed on the chest to obtain an ECG (an electrocardiogram; also abbreviated as EKG), which records the electrical activity of the heart. An ECG is useful when epilepsy is suspected because changes in heart rate or rhythm (which are reflected in the heart's electrical activity) often occur with seizures, and sometimes heart arrythmias can be a cause of provoked seizures.[63]

Electrodes may also be placed on the skin, over certain muscles (e.g., the neck, shoulders, limbs) to obtain a recording of the muscle's electrical activity. This is known as EMG (electromyography). EMG may help detect motor signs (i.e., muscle contractions) that may occur with seizures.[110,111]

4.3 Interpreting the EEG recording

Sometimes it's not enough to know what things mean, sometimes you have to know what things don't mean.
Bob Dylan

This section provides a brief explanation of the interpretation of an EEG recording. *Interpretation of an individual's EEG recording should be discussed with the medical professional.*

Interpreting the EEG patterns of brain wave activity is complex. Specially trained medical professionals interpret the recordings to discern normal and abnormal brain activity and identify seizure onset zones when possible. To the untrained eye, the EEG recording will appear as multiple wavy or pointed lines in rows. The different lines represent electrical activity in the areas of the brain that lie below the electrodes. By simultaneously graphing multiple lines, medical professionals can quickly compare activity in different areas of the brain. Interpreting EEG along with other factors (i.e., motor signs and nonmotor signs and symptoms) allows medical professionals to determine whether an individual is experiencing an epileptic seizure, provides information to help evaluate the risk of recurrence of epileptic seizures, and aids in diagnosing epilepsy. The use of automated systems and artificial intelligence to interpret EEG recordings is an area of active research.

EEG generates a recording of the electrical activity in groups of neurons close to the electrode. The electrodes closer to the region where the electrical activity occurs in the brain will record the most activity, potentially identifying the seizure onset zone, especially with focal onset seizures. In generalized seizures, electrical activity starts in both hemispheres, so a seizure onset zone is often not identifiable.

Important terms related to EEG interpretation include:

- **EEG wave:** Electrical activity in groups of neurons, captured by electrodes, and recorded on a graph. EEG waves have a peak (highest point), a trough (lowest point), and a baseline (middle point). EEG waves are classified primarily on amplitude and frequency:
    - **Amplitude:** The height of the EEG wave, which is the measure of the electric charge (i.e., the voltage) generated by the firing neurons.
    - **Frequency:** A measurement of how many EEG waves occur per second. EEG waves are named based on their typical frequency range (delta, theta, alpha, and beta are the most common).
- **EEG waveform:** Overall shape and pattern of the EEG waves and how they change over time. EEG waveforms may appear very regular and symmetrical, or they may have sharp rises or irregular patterns. Waveforms may be normal or abnormal, and what is considered normal varies with age, and some variation is expected, even in the absence of seizures. Waveforms may also be classified by amplitude and frequency (see above) and by shape and phase.
    - **Shape:** The overall appearance of the waveform; the edges of the lines can be described as spikes or more gradual sloping up and/or down. The shape of multiple EEG waves together is also considered, and specific patterns may be discerned.
    - **Phase:** A measurement of the timing relationship between different EEG waves (i.e., how areas of the brain synchronize with each other over time). Evaluation of the phase allows for comparison of different areas of the brain and can identify abnormalities.
- **Background:** Typical baseline brain wave activity when the brain is at rest.

- **Artifact:** An element of interference that shows up on an EEG recording due to something other than brain activity. Artifacts might be associated with eye blinks, muscle contractions, swallowing, or movement.[112]
- **Epileptic activity:** Abnormal electrical activity in the brain.
- **Epileptiform discharges:** Distinct EEG waveform patterns representative of epileptic activity. These may be further classified by their timing related to a seizure as:
  o **ictal epileptiform discharges** (occurring during the ictal phase of a seizure), or
  o **interictal epileptiform discharges** (occurring between seizures).

Recall that the activity of neurons and how they send messages to each other is what creates the electrical activity measured with EEG. Also recall the "all or none" concept, and that once the depolarization threshold has been reached, a neuron always fires with the same strength (amplitude). The only characteristic that changes is the frequency, or how often the neuron fires (i.e., a weak stimulus will result in slower firing or a lower frequency, and a strong stimulus will result in a quicker firing or a higher frequency). The number of neurons, how often they fire, and whether the messages are coordinated or uncontrolled will change what is shown on the EEG recording.

Despite the set amplitude reached when a single neuron fires, the EEG amplitude is variable because it represents the sum of multiple neurons firing at the same time.

To help understand this concept, think about a group of people who are all going to hit individual drums. Each person represents one neuron. Assume each drummer can only hit their drum with a consistent strength, just as a neuron can only fire with the same strength (amplitude). If all drummers hit their drums at the same time, the noise produced is louder than if they staggered their hits, even if they hit the drums with the same strength in both scenarios. It will be louder because the collective signal has a larger amplitude. In the same way, when multiple neurons fire at the same time, which can happen during a seizure, the EEG wave measured by an electrode will have a larger amplitude.

Recall that an electrode senses and records the electrical activity of a group of neurons close to the electrode, not just a single neuron. It is important to note that EEG only detects activity that occurs in groups of neurons in a place where the electrodes can sense the activity. In some cases, the electrical activity occurs deep in the brain and may not be detected by the surface electrodes.

The variability of the EEG amplitude creates waves, and the number of waves per second is known as the frequency of the electrical activity on EEG, which is related but different from the frequency at which a single neuron is discharging.

Figure 4.3.1 depicts a normal EEG recording without any seizure activity. In this figure, there are a few variations in the waveforms, but recall that normal brain waves have variations.

Recall that the main use of EEG in the diagnosis of epilepsy is to determine whether an individual is having an epileptic seizure or not, to evaluate the risk of recurrence of epileptic seizures in the future, and to aid in diagnosing epilepsy.

Two main EEG findings can lead to a diagnosis of epilepsy: seizures with epileptiform discharges and interictal epileptiform discharges.

- **Seizures with epileptiform discharges** are epileptic seizures characterized by organized epileptiform discharges, which are waveform patterns representative of epileptic activity. Epileptiform discharges are typically described as spikes, polyspikes, or spike-and-wave discharges, among others. These seizures recorded on EEG can be clinical seizures or electrographic seizures.
    - **Clinical seizures (also called electroclinical seizures)** are associated with obvious outward clinical changes, like motor signs and nonmotor signs and symptoms (i.e., absence or impaired consciousness).
    - **Electrographic seizures (also called subclinical seizures)** are seizures without clinical changes (no motor or nonmotor signs and symptoms, or impaired awareness), but with EEG changes showing organized, continuous, epileptiform discharges that in general last for more than 10 seconds and undergo at least a two-step evolution (each one-step evolution is defined by a change in shape, frequency, or location of the discharges). Individuals experiencing electrographic seizures will have no

change in level of awareness and will not know a seizure is occurring. These seizures may also occur in critically ill individuals who are in a coma.

- **Interictal epileptiform discharges** are epileptiform abnormalities observed on EEG between seizures without any clinical changes in the individual. Interictal epileptiform discharges are most often seen between seizures in someone with epilepsy. When interictal epileptiform discharges are abundant on EEG, it might lead to the diagnosis of epilepsy. Interictal epileptiform discharges might be seen with features specific to certain epilepsy syndromes, occurring with or without seizures. However, anyone might have *infrequent* interictal epileptiform discharges on EEG even if they do not have epilepsy or have not had a seizure. For these individuals, their risk for future seizures is the same as the general population, and the presence of these infrequent interictal epileptiform discharges does not indicate epilepsy.

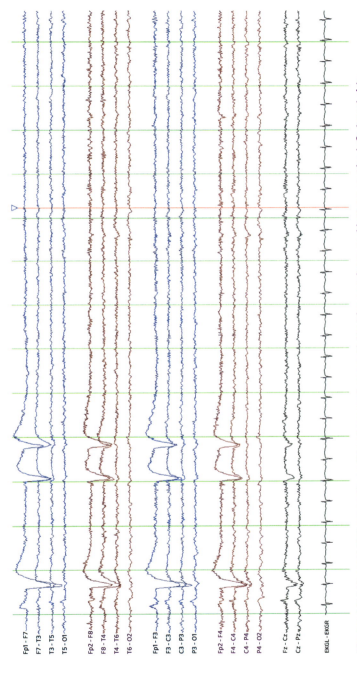

Figure 4.3.1 Normal EEG recording without any seizure activity. **The numbers and letters on the left-hand side** match the location of the electrodes. **The area between two green vertical lines** represents 1 second of time; the recording is 15 seconds long. **The blue and red horizontal lines** represent the brain wave activity in waveforms. The blue lines indicate activity occurring on the left half of the brain and the red on the right half of the brain. **The two black horizontal lines below the bottom red lines** indicate activity occurring in the middle of the brain. **The bottom black horizontal line** is the ECG/EKG recording. **The red vertical line** is the cursor and is not relevant.

4.4 Phases of a seizure and EEG

> You gain strength, courage and confidence by every experience in which you really stop to look fear in the face.
> **Eleanor Roosevelt**

The phases of a seizure may be observable by an onlooker, or they may be able to be seen only with EEG. Even with EEG, however, challenges exist in specifying the start and stop of specific seizure phases.

The phases were defined earlier in section 2.4. The following describes what is seen on an EEG recording for each seizure phase as depicted in Figure 4.4.1. Note that an additional phase, the interictal phase, is included here:

- **The preictal phase** may be characterized by changes in brain wave activity that indicate the onset of a seizure.
- **The ictal phase** is characterized by ictal epileptiform discharges, indicating a seizure.
- **The postictal phase** may show a rapid or gradual return to baseline brain wave activity.

- **The interictal phase** is the period *between* seizures in someone who has repeated seizures. Since the individual is not experiencing seizures during the interictal phase, they will display typical feelings and activities. However, on an EEG recording, the interictal phase may show abnormal brain waves, such as interictal epileptiform discharges. These commonly are present in individuals with epilepsy and may contribute to some cognitive and behavioral comorbidities, addressed in Chapter 9.[113,114] A particular type of abnormal activity seen on interictal EEG is hypsarrhythmia, which is characterized by a chaotic, irregular pattern of waveforms and is seen in individuals with epileptic spasms, particularly infantile spasms.[115]

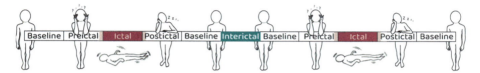

Figure 4.4.1 Seizure phases including the interictal phase between two seizures.

Figure 4.4.2 depicts an EEG recording of a focal seizure (ictal phase) in the right hemisphere, which progresses to a bilateral tonic-clonic seizure involving both hemispheres.

94 Epilepsy

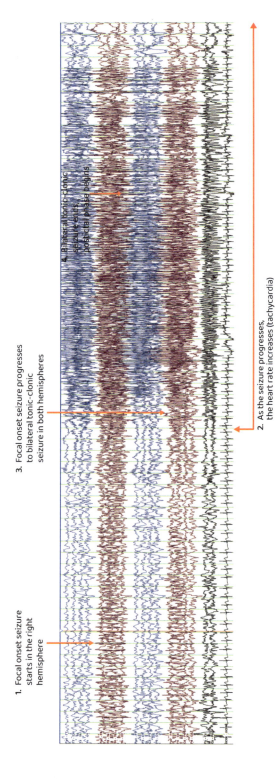

Figure 4.4.2 EEG recording of a focal seizure in the right hemisphere from onset (ictal phase) progressing to a bilateral tonic–clonic seizure involving both hemispheres. 1. The individual experiences a focal onset seizure depicted on the red horizontal line. 2. As the seizure progresses, the heart rate increases (tachycardia), as shown by shorter spacing between heart beats on the bottom black horizontal line. 3. The progression of the seizure is depicted in red and blue horizontal lines, indicating activity in both hemispheres. 4. The seizure ends, and the postictal phase begins.

4.5 Seizure recording and detection

*If you do not know where you are going,
every road will get you nowhere.*
Henry Kissinger

The unpredictable nature of epilepsy and the lack of control can negatively impact the quality of life for individuals with epilepsy. While EEG is a great tool to detect and record seizures, it is limited to doing so only during the test, which is a relatively small window of time. When seizures are accurately detected and recorded in a timely manner, seizure control may improve, and adverse events may decrease.[116,117] For instance, receiving a warning that a seizure is going to happen can allow the individual to remove themselves from an unsafe environment.

Other methods to record, detect, and predict seizures, including using technology or service animals, can offer individuals with epilepsy greater agency over the management of their condition.

Methods for recording seizures

Two methods for recording seizures include keeping a seizure diary and taking a video recording:

- **A seizure diary** can be kept by the individual with epilepsy, or by those observing the seizure. The details can be recorded in a journal, on a table or checklist, or even with a phone app. A seizure diary should include the characteristics of the seizure (including any auras), the date and time of the seizure, the length of time the seizure lasted, any triggers that led to the seizure, and any treatments or medications that were given and their effectiveness. A sample seizure diary is included in **Useful web resources.**
- **A video recording** with an in-home video recording system or phone camera may capture a seizure that can be reviewed later.

These methods have their limitations, however. Keeping a seizure diary can be inconvenient, and depending on the situation, it may be impossible to record a seizure. Someone who is experiencing a seizure with impaired awareness is not able to call for help when the seizure occurs or may not be able to recall the events of the seizure afterwards. Furthermore, nighttime seizures are often unnoticed, particularly in individuals who live alone. Studies have shown that seizure diaries are generally unreliable.[116]

Video recording will be helpful only if the seizure is a motor seizure and the individual is within the range of the video recording system at the time of the seizure. Using a phone camera may not be practical as anyone observing an individual having a seizure should focus on ensuring the individual's safety and providing care as needed, rather than trying to make a recording.

Seizure detection devices

Several seizure detection devices exist, and most work by recognizing typical changes in the body that are associated with seizures. These may include changes in heart rate or rhythm, temperature, motor activity, or sounds.[116] Some implanted devices (neuromodulation devices, described in Chapter 8) can detect brain electrical activity including seizures, although they do not currently provide real-time notification of a seizure occurring.

At the time of writing, the only available US FDA–cleared* seizure detection device is worn on the wrist and connects to a phone through an app (previously Embrace2 by Empatica, and now its successor EpiMonitor) (see Figure 4.5.1). EpiMonitor detects patterns associated with generalized tonic-clonic seizures, alerts caregivers with a GPS location, and monitors epilepsy, with the battery lasting up to seven days.

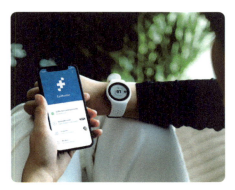
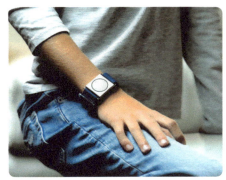

Figure 4.5.1 Seizure detection devices: Empatica and EpiMonitor (left) and Embrace2 (right). Reproduced with kind permission from Empatica.

Seizure detection devices have been shown to have benefits to users by providing a more comprehensive picture of the seizure activity to aid in better management. For example, they may provide more accurate timing of the seizure and allow evaluation of the circumstances when the seizure occurred. Wearable technology has been shown to decrease adverse events and injuries associated with seizures, such as prolonged apnea (periods when breathing stops) and SUDEP.[117] However, people with epilepsy will benefit from these technologies only if they are willing to use them, and for some they may be cost prohibitive. Individuals with epilepsy want such devices to be "attractive, comfortable, not obviously 'medical,' and to be highly usable and nonintrusive."[116] As well, seizure

---

* The US Food and Drug Administration (FDA) regulates food, drugs, and medical devices. FDA *clearance* for a medical device means the device is equivalent to another device that has been cleared or approved. FDA *approval* means that the benefits of the device in a particular population are found to outweigh potential side effects. International equivalents of the FDA exist in other countries.

detection devices may not detect generalized absence seizures or focal seizures without motor signs and symptoms.

At this point, seizure detection devices are viewed as a supplement to seizure diaries rather than a replacement. More research is needed to improve the devices, and more countries need to medically approve them and make them available.[116] Until then, a low- to no-cost option to detect generalized tonic-clonic seizures or focal motor seizures is to attach a small bell to the individual's limb (either a wrist or ankle for example). The sound of the bell can alert nearby caregivers of a seizure. This could be useful in a setting when someone isn't directly watching a child (e.g., when the child is playing in another room, or when the child is sleeping); the repeated ringing from a shaking limb could alert the caregiver.

Seizure response dogs and seizure predicting dogs

Dogs can be trained for both seizure response and seizure predicting to assist individuals with epilepsy.[118]

- Seizure response dogs may detect when a seizure is occurring and may be trained to bark or activate an alarm. They may also lie next to the individual who is having a seizure to comfort or protect them.
- Seizure predicting dogs have been reported to sense a change in an individual before a seizure occurs and may alert the person by certain behaviors such as making close eye contact, circling, pawing, or barking.[119] Even untrained dogs have been known to display certain patterns of behavior when seizures occur in individuals with epilepsy with whom they live.[120]

Studies have shown:

- Seizures may cause an individual to have a particular odor, and trained dogs have accurately discriminated between that odor and the odor of the same individual when they are not actively seizing.[121] In a group of trained dogs, a study found a 94 percent "probability of correctly distinguishing between ictal and interictal sweat samples."[122]

- Behavioral changes in dogs are noted before the onset of seizures, associated with preictal symptoms, and these behaviors positively influence the bond between the owner and the dog.[123]
- Improvements in reported quality of life factors such as independence, security, and self-confidence occur in individuals with epilepsy when matched with seizure response dogs compared to before owning the dog.[120]
- A device known as an accelerometer, which measures vibration and motion and is worn by a seizure predicting dog, may identify changes in behaviors of the dog, indicating an impending seizure in an individual with epilepsy. This can allow for real-time alerts to the individual or their caregiver.[118]

The use of seizure response dogs and seizure predicting dogs is not always an option, however. Training these dogs can take months to years, and the cost is often prohibitive. In addition, the relationship between the dog and the individual takes time to build, and the individual needs to be able to recognize the cues the dog provides, which can often be subtle. The needs of the dog also must be considered, and service dogs may become overly stressed in situations, which can impair the ability to be effective in the role.[119]

> Emma continued to have seizures in those first few months. She had outpatient EEGs and an overnight VEEG. We quickly learned that seizures aren't always as they are depicted in TV shows or movies. Epilepsy looks different for everyone, and some seizures can cause very little movement. Emma's seizures in the early days were mostly generalized tonic-clonic seizures, involving a lot of movement where both her arms and head would jerk, and her legs would become very spastic or stiff. She also often lost all control of her secretions and would drool a lot. We would need to put a towel next to her cheek just to help catch all the secretions. Emma's seizures often included breath-holding, leading to the color draining out of her face and her turning blue. As a parent, I found this so difficult to watch. I tried to remain calm, but that was easier said than done. Just when I was starting to think she was going to pass out, she would often take a big gasp of air. To this day, this is still how her seizures often present.

One morning in particular will never leave my memory. I went to her room to check on her to find her seizing badly. I ran over and picked her up and yelled for Scott to call 911. I knew by the puddle of drool that had formed on her bed sheet that she had been seizing for some time. The ambulance arrived and she continued to seize, even after getting to the hospital and after being given antiseizure medications.

In the rural area where we live, quick access to specialty pediatric care is a challenge. It was soon decided that Emma needed to be transferred by helicopter to the closest children's hospital. The doctors there estimated that she had been seizing for around 90 minutes and was in status epilepticus. She had to be sedated for over 24 hours to help calm her brain and stop the seizures.

When I think back to that day, I recall the kindness shown to me in that terrifying helicopter ride as I sat frozen in my seat sweating uncontrollably while feeling scared to death. I looked over at Emma, worried about how she was doing, and one of the medics placed her hand on my shoulder and said, "Don't worry. She's gonna be okay, mama!" It was just what I needed to hear. I will say that helicopter ride is something I hope to never, ever experience again.

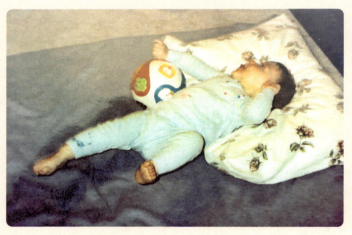

Emma at seven months.

4.5 SEIZURE RECORDING AND DETECTION

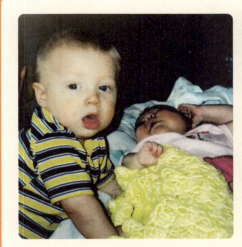 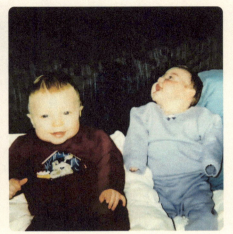

Jake (left) and Emma (right) at seven months.

Key points Chapter 4

- Electroencephalography, commonly known as EEG, measures and records the brain's electrical activity, generating a visual graph of brain waves.
- Video EEG (VEEG) involves the audiovisual recording of the individual while simultaneously measuring and recording brain wave activity. It is considered the gold standard for diagnosing epilepsy.
- During EEG, the medical professional evaluates the measured and recorded brain wave activity and observes the individual's level of awareness, motor signs, and nonmotor signs and symptoms.
- EEG records only live events, so it is possible that no events will occur while the individual is undergoing EEG. If certain triggers are identified for the individual, those triggers can be used to try to induce a seizure during EEG.
- A commonly used pattern of electrode placement is the International 10–20 system.
- The phases of a seizure may be observable by an onlooker or may only be seen with EEG. Challenges exist in specifying the start and stop of specific seizure phases.
- Methods to record seizures include using a seizure diary and video recording with an in-home video recording system or phone camera. These methods have their limitations.
- Several seizure detection devices exist, and most work by recognizing typical changes in the body that are associated with seizures. These may include changes in heart rate or rhythm, temperature, motor activity, or sounds.
- Dogs can be trained for seizure response or seizure prediction to assist individuals with epilepsy. Using seizure response dogs and seizure predicting dogs is not always an option. Training these dogs can take months to years, and the cost is often prohibitive.

Chapter 5

Diagnosis of epilepsy

Section 5.1 Introduction 105
Section 5.2 Brain imaging 106
Section 5.3 Laboratory tests 108
Section 5.4 Lumbar puncture 112
Section 5.5 Genetic testing 114
Key points Chapter 5 117

5.1 Introduction

When everything seems to be going against you, remember that the airplane takes off against the wind, not with it.

Henry Ford

Determining if an individual has epilepsy takes time and typically involves evaluating signs and symptoms of a seizure, and EEG, as first steps. While EEG is an extremely useful tool, it is only one test that medical professionals use to determine a diagnosis of epilepsy. Additional tests are often needed to differentiate epilepsy from other conditions, determine the epilepsy type and cause, and identify epilepsy syndromes and comorbidities. These tests may include:

- **Brain imaging**
- **Laboratory tests**
- **Lumbar puncture**
- **Genetic testing**

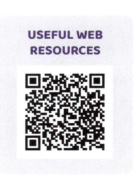

USEFUL WEB RESOURCES

5.2

Brain imaging

> Just because you're puzzled,
> doesn't mean life's jagged edges
> won't still fall into place for you.
> **Curtis Tyrone Jones**

Brain imaging is used to identify structural abnormalities in the brain, which may indicate a structural cause of epilepsy.[124] Structural abnormalities might include lesions due to trauma, lack of oxygen or nutrients, tumors, infections, autoimmune conditions, vascular disease, and genetic conditions. Some types of structural epilepsy, such as those caused by lesions or tumors, can be successfully treated with surgery to remove or shrink the area of abnormality.[32] After being removed, the tissue is examined to better identify the structural cause.

Brain imaging may be done with CT (computed tomography) and MRI (magnetic resonance imaging):

- **CT** uses radiation and identifies abnormalities or structural problems within the brain such as bleeding, cysts, tumors, or abnormally developed areas of the brain. A CT scan is usually more available than MRI, and it is remarkably faster, which makes it useful in urgent settings. A CT scan may be indicated after an MRI is done to check for specific findings, like calcium deposits (which may be related to rare conditions, including some that may cause epilepsy), since some findings may not be identified with MRI.[124] A notable risk of a CT scan is radiation exposure. Using the lowest radiation dose possible is recommended.[124]

- **MRI** does not use radiation; instead, magnetic force produces an enhanced picture of the brain and other soft tissue structures (e.g., nerves, vessels) that are not as visible on a CT scan.[124] The following specific types of MRI may be needed to evaluate for cardiovascular conditions (relating to the heart and blood vessels) or cerebrovascular conditions (relating to the brain and its blood vessels):
  - **Magnetic resonance angiogram (MRA):** This type of MRI is used to identify arteries (responsible for carrying oxygenated blood from the heart to the rest of the body, including the brain) and discern any that are malformed. These abnormalities may include obstruction to bloodflow, aneurysms (swelling of blood vessels), structural defects, or injuries to vessels.
  - **Magnetic resonance venogram (MRV):** This type of MRI is used to identify veins (responsible for carrying blood from all areas of the body, including the brain, back to the heart) and discern any that are malformed. These abnormalities may include blood clots, structural defects, or issues with bloodflow.

With both CT and MRI, contrast may be used. Contrast is a substance administered (often through an injection) to make internal organs and structures such as blood vessels show up better on medical imaging.

CT angiography is performed when vascular disease is suspected. It evaluates the arteries using contrast, and it is more sensitive than MRI or MRA for small arteries. CT contrast might cause allergic reactions, may affect kidney or thyroid function, and may interact with some medications (e.g., metformin, used to control blood sugar).

Contrast with MRI may be used to help enhance lesions, tumors, or brain abnormalities. MRI contrast might cause allergic reactions and may affect kidney or liver function.

5.3 Laboratory tests

Persistence and resilience only come from having been given the chance to work through difficult problems.
Gever Tulley

Typically, laboratory tests are done by taking a sample of body fluid or tissues (e.g., by drawing blood from a vein in the arm or obtaining a urine sample). The sample is evaluated, and the results are compared to typical ranges to determine whether the sample is within the typical range. Some laboratory tests may be used to rule out epilepsy, while others may be used to help confirm the diagnosis of epilepsy, including the type and cause.

Common laboratory tests used in the diagnosis of epilepsy include:

- **Prolactin levels**
- **Electrolyte levels**
- **Blood cell count**
- **Metabolism evaluation**
- **Autoimmune and immune dysregulation studies**
- **Toxicology screen**

Prolactin levels

Prolactin is a normally occurring hormone in the body, most often associated with milk production in lactating women (i.e., breastfeeding). However, some prolactin circulates in the blood in all individuals. Prolactin levels can be measured with a blood test, and prolactin has been found to be increased immediately following epileptic seizures, especially generalized tonic-clonic seizures.[125] While an elevated prolactin level is highly suggestive of an epileptic seizure (about 80 percent of events associated with elevated prolactin are actual epileptic seizures), it provides only one piece of information within the broader evaluation.[125] Prolactin is not routinely used in the diagnosis of epilepsy, but it may be useful in certain circumstances, especially when differentiating epileptic seizures from seizure mimics, such as PNES, or functional seizures.

Note that this test can be somewhat cumbersome as it involves going to a laboratory twice to have blood drawn: once within 10 to 20 minutes of the suspected seizure, *and* either prior to the suspected seizure or at least 24 hours after to obtain a baseline prolactin level.

Electrolyte levels

Common electrolytes are calcium, potassium, chloride, sodium, and magnesium, which are typically measured in blood and urine. Abnormal levels of electrolytes may help identify a metabolic cause of epilepsy or certain comorbidities. Abnormal levels may also lead to seizure mimics or provoked seizures, which can help rule out a diagnosis of epilepsy.[126]

Blood cell count

A complete blood count measures levels of blood components, including white blood cells, red blood cells, hemoglobin, and platelets. Levels that are outside the typical range may help identify comorbidities or an infectious cause of epilepsy.[127]

Metabolism evaluation

"Metabolism" refers to the chemical processes that help cells in the body convert food into energy.[128] A metabolic disorder is a disorder that affects the metabolism. An "inborn error of metabolism" is a metabolic disorder that is inherited and occurs before birth. However, metabolic disorders may also be acquired. Blood, urine, and cerebrospinal fluid* tests are used to evaluate metabolism and enzymes.†[129] Abnormal test results may indicate metabolic epilepsy.

Autoimmune and immune dysregulation studies

Autoimmune and immune dysregulation conditions occur when the immune system malfunctions, mistakenly attacking the body's own tissues or failing to regulate immune responses properly. Blood and cerebrospinal fluid tests are used to evaluate the presence of antibodies and immune markers. Abnormal levels may help identify an immune cause of epilepsy or of seizure mimics.

Toxicology screen

Toxins are poisonous substances. Toxins may be present in the body from the consumption of illicit drugs, certain plants or plant products, certain medications, or other chemicals.[130] A toxicology screen evaluates blood or urine for the presence of toxins. Some toxins may be a cause of provoked seizures, which can help rule out a diagnosis of epilepsy.

> During Emma's first year, it was a bit of a whirlwind with tests and doctor visits. When Emma was about eight months old, I took her to an appointment with a neurologist. I felt intimidated going to this appointment, fearing what the doctor would say about Emma. By the time I lugged her baby carrier, my purse, and a diaper bag in the middle of

---

* Cerebrospinal fluid is found within the brain and around the spinal cord. It helps protect the brain and spinal cord from injury.

† Enzymes are proteins that cause changes in cells or organs and support bodily functions.

winter through a parking ramp, up a flight of stairs, and off the elevator, I was sweating and disheveled, looking like I had been hit over the head with a frying pan and pushed out of a moving vehicle—not to mention sleep deprived and stressed out (remember, twins!). Everyone on the other side of that elevator door was dressed so nicely and professional looking. It was so quiet you could hear the clock ticking on the wall. I felt the tension in the air, and that lump in my throat was back again.

It was at this visit that I learned that my sweet Emma not only has epilepsy, she was also showing many signs of cerebral palsy. I didn't really understand that. I thought maybe it meant she would just have a little bit of cerebral palsy, not a lot, and that she would have some trouble walking. I think, reflecting on it, that was the neurologist's way of easing us into the diagnosis of yet another medical condition, one that would have a significant effect on Emma and her future.

The walls of the office were lined with an intimidating display of books and medical journals packed with all the information I needed to give me answers about Emma. I felt intimidated with the neurologist, too. I was just the mom; he was someone who knew everything there was to know about the brain and how it works. He oozed intelligence, and we were literally surrounded by this knowledge. But I have come to realize that no doctor, not even the smartest neurologist in the world, knows my daughter like I do. When it comes to Emma, I am the expert. And for those parents of a child with epilepsy who are reading this, you will be an expert too—even if you haven't read walls and walls of medical journals and books.

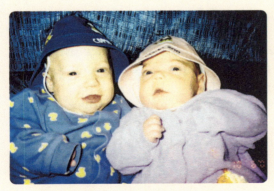

Jake (left) with Emma at six months.

5.4 Lumbar puncture

> Take a deep breath and do the difficult thing first.
> Mary Anne Radmacher

A lumbar puncture is a procedure in which a needle is inserted into the spinal column and a sample of cerebrospinal fluid is removed. The sample is evaluated in a laboratory to determine whether the components of the sample (e.g., appearance, cells, proteins) are within the typical range. Abnormal results can help differentiate epilepsy from other conditions, particularly provoked seizures from acute infectious causes. Abnormal results can also be used to help confirm a diagnosis of epilepsy, particularly epilepsy resulting from infectious or immune causes. Sedation or anesthesia may be required, especially in children, to ensure the individual remains still and comfortable during the procedure.

An individual undergoing a lumbar puncture is depicted in Figure 5.4.1.

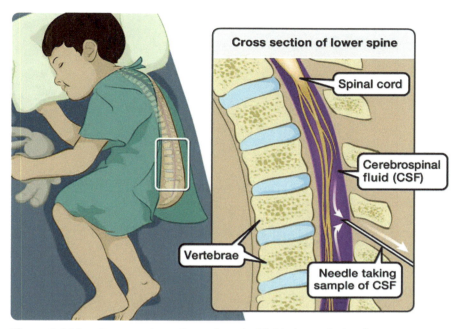

Figure 5.4.1 Lumbar puncture. Reproduced with kind permission from AboutKidsHealth. © 2004–2024 AboutKidsHealth.

5.5

Genetic testing

> There's as many atoms in a single molecule of your DNA
> as there are stars in the typical galaxy.
> We are, each of us, a little universe.
>
> **Neil deGrasse Tyson**

Genetic testing may be used to determine the cause and type of epilepsy, identify epilepsy syndromes, or evaluate for the presence of comorbidities. Genetic testing can help guide epilepsy management.

"Genes" are the units of heredity transferred from parent to offspring. "Genetics" is a branch of science that studies genes or heredity. The building blocks of genes are contained in DNA in the form of a genetic "code," which provides instructions for the gene.[16] Alterations in the genetic code, such as a mutation in a particular gene, a duplication of a gene, or a deletion of a gene, can cause epilepsy. Some comorbidities are also associated with alterations in genes.

Figure 5.5.1 presents a simple graphic explanation of heredity. It shows one parent (the dad) who has a condition associated with a gene with a mutation—a "nonworking" gene, designated with an "x." Because just one of the parents has this gene, the odds of the child inheriting it, and therefore having the condition, are 50 percent. This is shown in the figure, with two of the four children having the condition. But it could have turned out that all the children inherited the gene—or none of them. Each child, individually, that this couple has will have the same 50 percent chance of inheriting the condition.

This inheritance pattern is termed autosomal dominant inheritance pattern, which some types of epilepsy and epilepsy syndromes follow. That means that if a person has just one copy of the nonworking gene, they will have the condition.

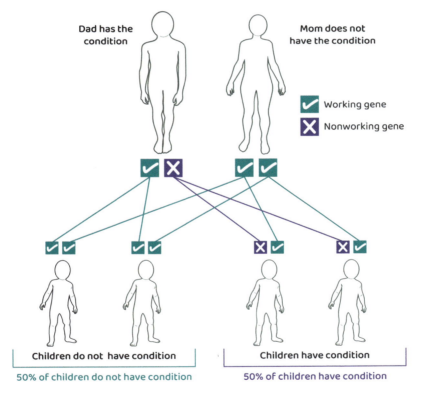

Figure 5.5.1 Autosomal dominant inheritance pattern from parents to children. Adapted with kind permission from Genetic Support Foundation.

The autosomal dominant pattern is one pattern of inheritance, but different patterns exist. And even though the epilepsy cause (or epilepsy syndrome) is identified as genetic, it does not necessarily mean that epilepsy has been inherited. When a mutation appears spontaneously in a gene for the first time in children but is not present in either parent, it is known as a *de novo* mutation. *De novo* mutations are a significant contributor to genetic causes of epilepsy and epilepsy syndromes. This new mutated gene can then be passed onto future children.

Therefore, epilepsy with a genetic cause can be either inherited or spontaneously appear. Ascertaining which is helpful for parents planning to have children, if one parent has epilepsy with a genetic cause. It can also be helpful to the individual with epilepsy with a genetic cause or their family members for understanding the potential risk of passing along a specific genetic epilepsy.[131]

Genetic testing involves examining the DNA in blood, body fluids (usually saliva), or tissue samples. If a family chooses to have genetic testing, it is recommended that they have it done in a center offering genetic counseling to help interpret and discuss the results.[132]

While genetic testing may establish if there is a genetic cause of epilepsy or any comorbidities, it has limitations. First, it may not be practical or possible depending on geographic location or cost. As well, it may reveal other conditions or potential risks for other conditions not related to epilepsy, which can generate undue anxiety or stress. In that case, the family might opt to have only the information that is related to the epilepsy diagnosis disclosed at the time of testing. However, despite these limitations, genetic testing can be helpful in research, clinical trials, and future treatments under investigation.

More information on genetic testing and epilepsy is included in Appendix 5 (online).

Key points Chapter 5

- While EEG is an extremely useful tool, it is only one test that medical professionals use to determine a diagnosis of epilepsy.
- Additional tests are often needed to differentiate epilepsy from other conditions, determine the epilepsy type and cause, and identify epilepsy syndromes and comorbidities. These may include brain imaging, laboratory tests, lumbar puncture, and genetic testing.
- Brain imaging is used to identify structural abnormalities in the brain, which may indicate a structural cause of epilepsy.
- Some laboratory tests may be used to rule out epilepsy, while others may be used to help confirm the diagnosis of epilepsy, including the type and cause.
- A lumbar puncture is a procedure in which a needle is inserted into the spinal column and a sample of cerebrospinal fluid is removed. Abnormal results can help differentiate epilepsy from other conditions, particularly provoked seizures from acute infectious causes. Abnormal results can also be used to help confirm a diagnosis of epilepsy, particularly epilepsy resulting from infectious or immune causes.
- Genetic testing may be used to determine the cause and type of epilepsy, identify epilepsy syndromes, or evaluate for the presence of comorbidities. Genetic testing can help guide epilepsy management.

Chapter 6

Causes of epilepsy

Section 6.1 Introduction 121

Section 6.2 Structural 123

Section 6.3 Genetic 125

Section 6.4 Infectious 127

Section 6.5 Metabolic 129

Section 6.6 Immune 131

Section 6.7 Unknown 133

Key points Chapter 6 135

6.1 Introduction

> If you know the why,
> you can live any how.
> **Friedrich Nietzsche**

The cause of a condition is known as the etiology.[133] Figure 6.1.1 depicts the framework for classification of epilepsy. Causes (etiologies) of epilepsy are shown in the right-hand column.

The causes of epilepsy are the same as the causes of unprovoked seizures detailed in section 1.2: structural, genetic, infectious, metabolic, and immune. The cause may also be unknown, which is the case in about 50 percent of epilepsy worldwide.[24] An individual may also have multiple causes of epilepsy. Determining the cause, when possible, helps guide management and can provide clues to long-term prognosis.[134]

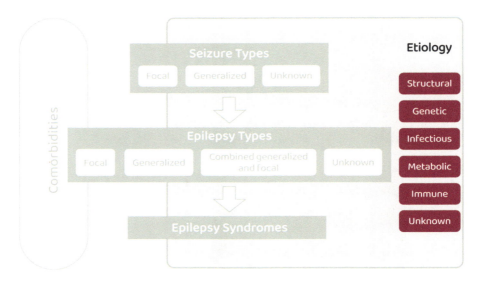

Figure 6.1.1 ILAE framework for classifying epilepsy. Adapted from *Epilepsia*, a journal of the ILAE. Used under a Creative Commons Attribution-Sharealike 4.0 International License https://creativecommons.org/licenses/by-sa/4.0/

EEG is a diagnostic test for anyone with suspected epilepsy, and it can help identify seizure onset zone, seizure type, and epilepsy type, which are useful in further determining the cause of epilepsy. The cause can then be identified with additional tests.

The following sections address each cause:

- **Structural**
- **Genetic**
- **Infectious**
- **Metabolic**
- **Immune**
- **Unknown**

In each section, the tests used to help determine the cause, in addition to EEG, are outlined.

USEFUL WEB RESOURCES

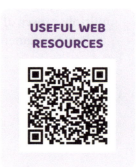

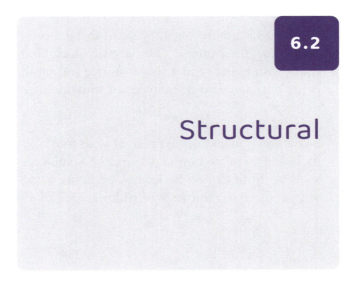

6.2

Structural

Don't be pushed around by the fears in your mind.
Be led by the dreams in your heart.
Roy T. Bennett

Epilepsy can be caused by a distinct structural abnormality (i.e., anatomical) in the brain; this is known as structural epilepsy. A structural cause of epilepsy may be either congenital or acquired:

- Congenital abnormalities are those that are present from birth and include structural abnormalities and atypical brain development.
- Acquired abnormalities are those that are not present from birth; they are acquired due to an event that occurs at or after the time of birth. Acquired structural causes include trauma, bleeding, lesions (abnormal tissue), infections, tumors, strokes, or scarring from anoxic (lack of oxygen) events.

Hippocampal sclerosis is the most common structural abnormality associated with focal epilepsy and the most common abnormality found in individuals with temporal lobe epilepsy, especially medial temporal lobe epilepsy.[131,135] Tumors are a structural abnormality that causes focal onset seizures and accounts for 0.2 to 6.0 percent of all child-onset epilepsy and 10 to 15 percent of adult-onset epilepsy.[131]

In both low- and high-income countries, structural causes of epilepsy are common, but they seem to be more common in low-income countries. For example, 59 percent of children age one month to 16 years with epilepsy in a low-resource setting in India have a structural cause compared to 37 percent of individuals of all ages with epilepsy in Norway.[131,136,137]

Structural epilepsy often presents with focal onset seizures but may also include generalized onset seizures.[138] Some types of structural epilepsy, such as those caused by lesions or tumors, can be successfully treated with surgery to remove or shrink the area of abnormality.[32]

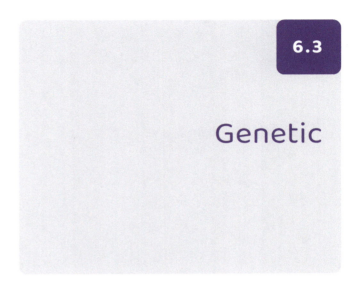

6.3

Genetic

> If there's a single lesson that life teaches us, it's that wishing doesn't make it so.
> **Lev Grossman**

Epilepsy can be caused by or closely associated with changes in genes; this is known as genetic epilepsy. A genetic cause of epilepsy may be inherited or spontaneously occur as a new gene mutation (*de novo*). Many epilepsy syndromes have a genetic cause.[139] In both low- and high-income countries, a genetic cause accounts for approximately 20 to 32 percent of all epilepsy cases in children and adults.[22,136,137,140]

Genetic epilepsy may be identified with genetic testing (see section 5.5). However, genetic testing may not identify the gene mutation. The medical professional may suspect that the individual has a *presumed* genetic epilepsy, particularly if there is a family history of epilepsy.[140]

Genetic epilepsy can present with any seizure type and is often suspected when epilepsy develops very early in life.[141] Some types of genetic epilepsy are associated with specific seizure types. Genetic epilepsy is most often treated with antiseizure medication or with the ketogenic diet.[141] Some gene therapy treatments are currently under development and might be clinically available in the coming years.

6.4 Infectious

> I can't change the direction of the wind, but I can adjust my sails to always reach my destination.
> **Jimmy Dean**

Epilepsy can be caused by a previous (not acute) brain infection; this is known as infectious epilepsy. Acute infections of the brain, such as meningitis or encephalitis, may cause provoked seizures.[15] (Meningitis involves inflammation of the membranes—the meninges—surrounding the brain and spinal cord. Encephalitis involves inflammation of the brain tissue itself.) In the acute stage, these seizures are *not* diagnosed as infectious epilepsy and do *not* typically persist after the infection is treated.[15] However, if seizures persist after the acute infectious period (i.e., after one to two weeks) and lead to epilepsy, the cause of the epilepsy is termed infectious.[15,22,142]

Infectious epilepsy is more common in low-income countries where there are higher rates of infections associated with lack of resources such as vaccinations, clean water, and sanitation.[143] For example, 26 percent of individuals of all ages with epilepsy in sub-Saharan Africa have an infectious cause compared to only 6 percent of individuals of all ages with epilepsy in Norway.[137,144] Infections such as cerebral malaria, tuberculosis, HIV, cytomegalovirus, cerebral toxoplasmosis, and neurocysticercosis* contribute to infectious epilepsy.[32,81,131] Infectious epilepsy may be preventable with appropriate hygiene measures, vaccinations, and treatment of infections.[145]

Taking a medical history, including recent or previous infections, is important and may be enough to identify an infectious cause of epilepsy. Additional testing such as MRI, lumbar puncture, or other laboratory tests may also be performed.[32] A specific laboratory test, clinical metagenomic sequencing, can detect genetic material causing the infection and may also confirm a previous infection.[146] Sometimes a laboratory evaluation of the immune system is needed to identify an immune deficiency that may have predisposed the individual to develop an infection that reached the brain.

Sometimes, infectious epilepsy may also be structural epilepsy when infections cause structural abnormalities in the brain.[15] In these cases, the abnormality may be surgically removed.

Infectious epilepsy can present with different types of seizures. If a structural abnormality has resulted from the infection, the seizure type will depend on the location of the abnormality. Further, infectious epilepsy can be drug resistant, especially when it results in structural abnormalities.[142]

---

* These infections typically occur in the brain or are systemic (occur throughout the body) and are caused by bacteria, viruses, or parasites.

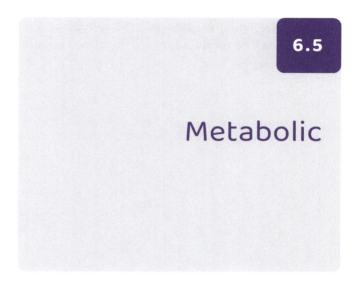

6.5 Metabolic

> You never know how strong you are until being strong is your only choice.
> **Bob Marley**

Epilepsy can be caused by a metabolic disorder; this is known as metabolic epilepsy. Metabolic disorders may be either inborn (inherited) errors of metabolism or acquired due to environmental conditions such as exposure to toxins or dietary deficiencies.[147] Several types of metabolic epilepsy exist, and many epilepsy syndromes have a metabolic cause.[148] Metabolic causes are less common than other causes, accounting for only 1 to 2 percent of epilepsy in children and adults, regardless of the income status of the country.[131,136]

Metabolic causes of epilepsy are often identified with laboratory testing of blood, urine, cerebrospinal fluid, or other tissues.[149] Metabolic epilepsy may be suspected in infants or children who have both epilepsy and issues with food intake (either due to intolerance or aversion) or failure to thrive.[148]

Metabolic epilepsy can present with any type of seizure. However, specific types of metabolic epilepsy are often accompanied by specific types of seizures. Antiseizure medications may be ineffective in managing metabolic epilepsy. Instead, the ketogenic diet, vitamins, or supplements may be used to provide improved seizure control.[147,148,150]

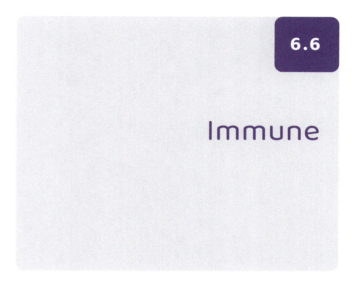

6.6 Immune

> What is now proved was once only imagin'd.
> **William Blake**

Epilepsy can be caused by an alteration in the body's defense system (immune system) against infections; this is known as immune epilepsy. Epilepsy with an immune cause may also be termed autoimmune epilepsy or immune-mediated epilepsy when the immune system begins to attack normal, healthy cells, leading to inflammation in the brain that results in epilepsy.[15,142] Epilepsy syndromes may also have an immune cause.

Immune epilepsy is a field of active research, and the rate of immune causes of epilepsy is difficult to measure.[151,152] Immune causes of epilepsy are often identified by laboratory testing of blood or cerebrospinal fluid to evaluate specific antibodies.[32,81] Brain imaging, such as MRI, may also be needed.[32,149]

Immune epilepsy often presents with focal onset seizures, which may be drug resistant.[32] Focal onset seizures may also evolve into bilateral tonic-clonic seizures. Antiseizure medications are more effective when used alongside immunotherapies for immune epilepsy.[152] The administration of steroids may also be considered.

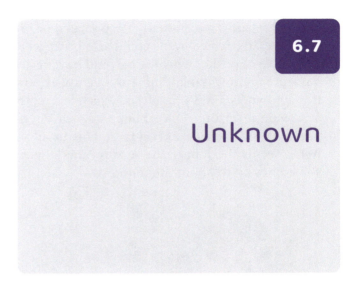

6.7 Unknown

Somewhere, something incredible is waiting to be known.
Carl Sagan

Epilepsy with an unknown cause is common; about 50 percent of epilepsy cases worldwide are classified as unknown.[24] Often, the cause of the epilepsy is found only with additional testing (e.g., brain imaging, laboratory tests, genetic testing) that is not available in all parts of the world, which may be the reason for the number of unknown epilepsy cases.

Individuals with unknown epilepsy should be reevaluated regularly (about every one to two years). Epilepsy with an unknown cause may also be reclassified with later research and medical advances.

Since Emma was diagnosed with a brain bleed shortly after birth, this was quickly labeled as the cause of her epilepsy (structural).

Emma's seizures were usually sleep related or brought on by the occasional fever. Extreme fatigue could also bring on a seizure, but sometimes it was the opposite, where she would have rested and then would have a seizure upon waking. Emma frequently experiences a postictal condition known as Todd's paralysis, which is a temporary state of paralysis following a seizure. Once Emma's seizure is over, she has temporary paralysis on one side of her face. This usually passes quickly for her, but it seems the longer the seizure, the longer the paralysis will last, sometimes up to about 30 minutes.

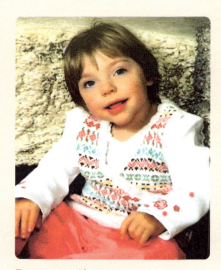

Emma, age three.

Key points Chapter 6

- The causes of epilepsy include structural, genetic, infectious, metabolic, and immune. The cause may also be unknown; this accounts for about 50 percent of epilepsy cases worldwide.
- Structural epilepsy is caused by a distinct structural abnormality of the brain.
- Structural epilepsy often presents with focal onset seizures but may also include generalized onset seizures.
- Some types of structural epilepsy, such as those caused by lesions or tumors, can be successfully treated with surgery to remove or shrink the area of abnormality.
- Genetic epilepsy is caused by or closely associated with changes in genes.
- Genetic epilepsy can present with any seizure type and is often suspected when epilepsy develops very early in life.
- Genetic epilepsy is most often treated with antiseizure medication or with a ketogenic diet.
- Infectious epilepsy occurs due to a previous (not acute) brain infection.
- Infectious epilepsy can present with different types of seizures. Infectious epilepsy can be drug resistant, especially when it results in structural abnormalities.
- Metabolic epilepsy is caused by a metabolic disorder. Metabolic disorders may either be inborn (inherited) errors of metabolism or acquired due to environmental conditions such as exposure to toxins or dietary deficiencies.
- Metabolic epilepsy can present with any type of seizure. However, specific types of metabolic epilepsy are often accompanied by specific types of seizures.
- Antiseizure medications may be ineffective in managing metabolic epilepsy. Instead, a ketogenic diet, vitamins, or supplements may be used to provide improved seizure control.
- Immune epilepsy is caused by an alteration in the body's defense system (immune system) against infections.
- Immune epilepsy often presents with focal onset seizures, which may be drug resistant. Focal onset seizures may also evolve into bilateral tonic-clonic seizures.

- Antiseizure medications are more effective when used alongside immunotherapies for immune epilepsy. The administration of steroids may also be considered.

Chapter 7

Epilepsy syndromes

Section 7.1 Introduction 139
Section 7.2 Onset in the neonatal period and infancy 142
Section 7.3 Onset in childhood 149
Section 7.4 Onset in adolescence and adulthood 154
Section 7.5 Onset at a variable age 157
Key points Chapter 7 159

7.1 Introduction

> Because learning does not consist only of knowing
> what we must or we can do, but also of knowing
> what we could do and perhaps should not do.
> **Umberto Eco**

An epilepsy syndrome is a group of symptoms that consistently occur together and are associated with the diagnosis of epilepsy. A more formal definition is "a characteristic cluster of clinical and EEG features, often supported by specific etiological findings (structural, genetic, metabolic, immune, and infectious)."[7] Identifying the epilepsy syndrome can often be more important than identifying the cause of epilepsy for deciding management, which makes this step of the diagnostic journey very important. Furthermore, identifying the epilepsy syndrome helps identify comorbidities earlier and helps determine long-term prognosis.

Within the ILAE framework for classifying epilepsy (Figure 7.1.1), identifying syndromes is the final step in diagnosing epilepsy in an individual. Some individuals diagnosed with epilepsy will not have an identified epilepsy syndrome, so the epilepsy type (focal, generalized, combined generalized and focal, or unknown) may be the final step in their epilepsy diagnosis. Sometimes, an epilepsy syndrome may be identified years later due to the progression of epilepsy in the individual, new research, and/or further testing.

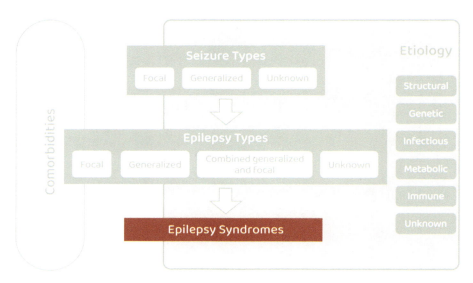

Figure 7.1.1 ILAE framework for classifying epilepsy. Adapted from *Epilepsia*, a journal of the ILAE. Used under a Creative Commons Attribution-Sharealike 4.0 International License https://creativecommons.org/licenses/by-sa/4.0/

Epilepsy syndromes are identified at variable ages—from the neonatal period to adulthood—but more commonly when the onset of epilepsy is in the neonatal period, infancy, or childhood. Fifty-four percent of children with epilepsy under the age of three have an identified epilepsy syndrome,[153] compared to 28 to 29 percent of children with epilepsy of all ages.[154] Some epilepsy syndromes may be outgrown in infancy or childhood, while others may persist into adulthood.

Sometimes individuals who have an epilepsy syndrome associated with onset at one age may later develop another epilepsy syndrome associated with onset at a later age. For example, about 30 percent of individuals with West syndrome (an epilepsy syndrome associated with onset in infancy) later develop Lennox-Gastaut syndrome (an epilepsy syndrome associated with onset in childhood).[139]

Epilepsy syndromes may be identified by characteristics including the age of epilepsy onset, seizure type, cause, and developmental impact:

- **Age of epilepsy onset:** This is the main way in which the syndromes are classified.
- **Seizure type:** This identifies the predominant seizure type.
- **Cause:** This includes structural, genetic, infectious, metabolic, immune, or unknown causes. Epilepsy syndromes frequently have a genetic cause, which is associated with a known gene mutation, although the cause varies by individual.[139]
- **Developmental impact:** Many epilepsy syndromes impact developmental milestones (key skills or abilities achieved by children at certain ages in areas including physical, cognitive, social, and emotional development). When children fall outside the typical age range for reaching these milestones, they may be diagnosed with a developmental delay.[155] Developmental delay is a common comorbidity of epilepsy and is addressed in Chapter 9.

Epilepsy syndromes are classified by age of onset:

- **Onset in the neonatal period and infancy**
- **Onset in childhood**
- **Onset in adolescence and adulthood**
- **Onset at a variable age**

This chapter includes a list of the syndromes in each age group. Within each age group, select syndromes are described in more detail. Information about the other syndromes is available in Appendix 6 (online).

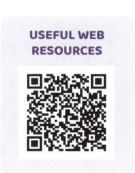

USEFUL WEB RESOURCES

7.2 Onset in the neonatal period and infancy

Stories are like children. They grow in their own way.
Madeleine L'Engle

The neonatal period is defined as the first 28 days of life. Infancy is the first year of life. Epilepsy syndromes with onset in this age group include:

- Self-limited epilepsy syndromes
- Developmental and epileptic encephalopathies (DEEs)
- Etiology-specific syndromes

Self-limited epilepsy syndromes

"Self-limited" refers to a condition that spontaneously resolves.[15,58] Self-limited epilepsy syndromes with onset in the neonatal period and infancy occur in otherwise healthy neonates and infants with typical development. Results of physical examinations, laboratory tests, brain imaging, and interictal EEG are typically normal. Most often, pregnancy and birth history are unremarkable.[139] These syndromes have a genetic cause, but a family history of the syndrome may or may not be present; many of the mutations arise *de novo*. These syndromes are typically responsive to antiseizure medications.[139] They resolve at predictable ages and are typically outgrown in infancy or childhood, although some individuals will develop another epilepsy syndrome.

Self-limited epilepsy syndromes with onset in the neonatal period and infancy include:

- Self-limited neonatal seizures and self-limited familial* neonatal epilepsy (SeLNE)
- Self-limited familial infantile epilepsy and self-limited infantile epilepsy (SeLIE)
- Genetic epilepsy with febrile seizures plus (GEFS+)
- Myoclonic epilepsy in infancy

Developmental and epileptic encephalopathies

Developmental and epileptic encephalopathies (DEEs) are epilepsy syndromes that are associated with developmental delay and cognition issues in which the developmental impairment *and* the epileptic activity contribute to the outcome. With DEEs, frequent seizures or interictal epileptiform discharges (observed on EEG) may influence the developmental delay.[156,157] The developmental delay may correlate with the age of onset of epilepsy, with the developmental delay usually becoming evident in infancy or childhood.[157]

DEEs with onset in the neonatal period and infancy begin sometime in the first year of life and are not self-limited (i.e., they do not resolve). DEEs are characterized by developmental delay and may have other associated comorbidities. Results of physical examinations are often atypical, and abnormal tone, posture, or movement may be evident.[139] Interictal EEG is abnormal and laboratory tests or brain imaging may be used to identify the cause.[139] Seizures may be very difficult to control and may be drug resistant.[139]

---

* In the case of self-limited familial epilepsy syndromes, a family history always exists. If no family history can be identified, the syndrome is known as a self-limited epilepsy syndrome (i.e., removing the term "familial").

DEEs with onset in the neonatal period and infancy include:

- Infantile epileptic spasms syndrome (West syndrome)
- Dravet syndrome (previously known as severe myoclonic epilepsy of infancy)
- Early-infantile epileptic encephalopathy (Ohtahara syndrome or early myoclonic encephalopathy)
- Epilepsy of infancy with migrating focal seizures

Two DEEs with onset in the neonatal period and infancy are West syndrome and Dravet syndrome, which are described in detail below. Expanded information about the other syndromes with onset in the neonatal period and infancy is available in Appendix 6 (online).

a) Infantile epileptic spasms syndrome (West syndrome)

Infantile epileptic spasms syndrome (IESS), or West syndrome, typically presents between 3 and 12 months of age, and developmental progress prior to the onset is often normal, with developmental delays emerging over time and intellectual disability resulting in most individuals.[139,158,159] This syndrome is characterized by epileptic spasms ranging from a few to over a hundred in clusters while awake or during sleep. In some instances, focal seizures may also occur at the beginning or end of the spasms.[158] In 30 percent of individuals, the cause is structural, but it may also be genetic or metabolic.[115] If the cause is genetic, IESS syndrome is rarely inherited, with *de novo* mutations being more typical. Individuals with this syndrome often develop other epilepsy syndromes as well.[139]

Comorbidities such as Down syndrome and tuberous sclerosis are often associated with IESS/West syndrome, and individuals may also develop autism spectrum disorder.[159] Management typically includes antiseizure medications and ACTH (adrenocorticotropic hormone therapy).[160] The ketogenic diet may also be considered.[161]

b) Dravet syndrome

Dravet syndrome (previously known as severe myoclonic epilepsy of infancy) presents within the first year of life with developmental delays beginning after the onset of seizures and typically apparent by three years of age.[139,162] Febrile seizures are often the first seizure, and seizures may also be triggered by vaccines, flashing lights, or stress.[162,163] Dravet syndrome is characterized by focal, focal to bilateral tonic-clonic seizures, and generalized seizures that are often prolonged and may lead to status epilepticus.[163] Myoclonic and absence seizures may also occur, and drug-resistant, lifelong seizures often develop.[163]

Dravet syndrome is often caused by a genetic mutation in the *SCN1A* gene. This may be due to a *de novo* mutation or be inherited; 30 to 50 percent of those diagnosed with Dravet syndrome have a family history of seizures.[162]

Comorbidities are common and often include movement and sleep disorders.[7] Management of Dravet syndrome includes antiseizure medications such as fenfluramine, stiripentol, cannabidiol (an antiseizure medication derived from the cannabis plant, known as medical cannabis), or the ketogenic diet.[164,165]

Etiology-specific epilepsy syndromes

Etiology-specific epilepsy syndromes have a well-defined cause. It may be structural, genetic, infectious, metabolic, or immune, although genetic and metabolic causes are the most common. Etiology-specific epilepsy syndromes present with consistent characteristics, including seizure type, impacted gene and inheritance pattern (when genetic), developmental impact, and comorbidities.[139] In addition, specific EEG findings, brain imaging results, and response to management are consistent.

Some etiology-specific epilepsy syndromes also include "DEE" in the name of the syndrome, referring to the developmental epileptic encephalopathy that accompanies it. If the etiology is not yet known, the syndrome may be identified as a DEE (as above), but when the etiology is known, it is better identified as an etiology-specific epilepsy syndrome. Seizures are often drug resistant and antiseizure medication may not work. Effective management may include special diets, surgery, or medications (other than antiseizure medications, such as steroids).

Etiology-specific epilepsy syndromes with onset in the neonatal period and infancy include:

- Sturge-Weber syndrome
- KCNQ2 DEE
- Pyridoxine dependent (ALDH7A1)-DEE (PD-DEE) and pyridox-(am)ine-5'-phosphate deficiency (PNPO)-DEE (P5PD-DEE)
- CDKL5-DEE
- PCDH19 clustering epilepsy
- Glucose transporter protein type 1 deficiency syndrome (GLUT1-DS)
- Gelastic seizures with hypothalamic hamartoma

Sturge-Weber syndrome is one etiology-specific epilepsy syndrome with onset in the neonatal period and infancy and is described in detail below. Expanded information about the other etiology-specific syndromes with onset in the neonatal period and infancy is available in Appendix 6 (online).

Sturge-Weber syndrome is present at birth with seizures typically beginning within the first six months of life. Developmental delay is common.[166] Sturge-Weber syndrome is characterized by focal seizures, focal to bilateral tonic-clonic seizures, epileptic spasms, and status epilepticus. However, seizures are present only in 75 to 90 percent of all individuals with this syndrome, with some individuals never having a seizure.[167] Structural or genetic causes have been noted with genetic causes typically due to *de novo* mutations and not inherited.[167]

Angiomas (lesions caused by atypical growth of blood vessels) may be present in the brain, in the eye, and as capillary malformations on the face. When these appear on the face, they are called port-wine stains. Stroke-like events resulting in hemiparesis (weakness or partial paralysis on one side of the body) may occur.[166] Management of Sturge-Weber syndrome may include antiseizure medications or epilepsy surgery if drug-resistant seizures develop. The ketogenic diet may also be used.[139] Low-dose aspirin beginning in infancy may be given to prevent stroke-like events.[166]

When Emma was about a year old, she developed a kind of seizure we had not seen before. She would be lying on her back and, at the same time, both arms would come up to her chest level and make a quick sweeping motion to the right side, almost like what someone directing traffic would do. These motions were quick, concise, and happened in repeated clusters. I called the neurologist (who, by then, I had on speed dial), who told us to bring her to the hospital. There, the doctors observed the same movement and identified them as infantile spasms, and Emma was eventually diagnosed with West syndrome. We were presented with two treatment options. One was to do a daily injection of a medication known as ACTH. The second was a new treatment that was still somewhat experimental without the solid track record of ACTH. I didn't want to take a chance on something that may not work when the neurologist seemed to think ACTH would definitely work. This brought to us the world of ACTH injections. I will say now, as a parent, you have no idea what you're capable of until it's staring you in the face and your child's life depends on it. Giving my own sweet baby a shot in the thigh every morning was not exactly a happy memory and certainly not something I envisioned in my parenting journey. I was so worried I might do something wrong. What if I put the needle in too fast or too slow? I remember feeling so bad about hurting her. However, like parents do, I stepped up and decided I had to do this for her no matter how difficult it was for me.

The injections worked well and stopped the infantile spasms. But she did develop a "moon face," which is one of the side effects of ACTH, due to the added weight and swelling of the face, in particular.

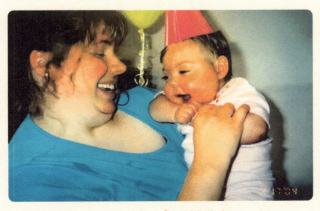

Anna, holding Emma at her first birthday party.

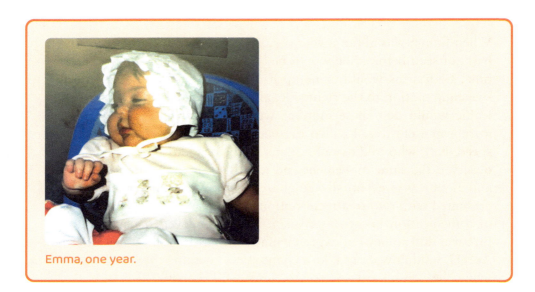

Emma, one year.

7.3

Onset in childhood

Anyone who does anything to help a child in his life is a hero to me.
Fred Rogers

Childhood is defined as the period between infancy and adolescence (age one to nine). Epilepsy syndromes with onset in this age group include:

- **Self-limited focal epilepsy syndromes**
- **Developmental and epileptic encephalopathies (DEEs)**
- **Generalized epilepsy syndromes**

Self-limited focal epilepsy syndromes

Recall that "self-limited" refers to a condition that spontaneously resolves. Self-limited focal epilepsy syndromes are characterized by focal seizures that may be infrequent or sporadic and may progress to generalized seizures. Seizures often respond well to antiseizure medications and, in many cases, the antiseizure medication may be stopped.[168] These syndromes are typically outgrown by puberty or early adulthood, although some individuals will develop another epilepsy syndrome.

Those with self-limited focal epilepsy syndromes with onset in childhood usually have typical development without comorbidities, but some challenges with language, learning, and behavior may exist during periods of seizures, then resolve. Self-limited focal epilepsy syndromes with onset in childhood include:

- Self-limited epilepsy with centrotemporal spikes (SeLECTs) (previously known as Rolandic epilepsy)
- Self-limited epilepsy with autonomic seizures (SeLEAS) (previously known as Panayiotopoulos syndrome)
- Childhood occipital visual epilepsy (COVE)
- Photosensitive occipital lobe epilepsy (POLE)

Developmental and epileptic encephalopathies

Recall that developmental and epileptic encephalopathies (DEEs) are epilepsy syndromes that are associated with developmental delay and cognition issues in which the developmental impairment *and* the epileptic activity contribute to the outcome. With DEEs, frequent seizures or interictal epileptiform discharges (observed on EEG) may influence the developmental delay.[156,157] The developmental delay may correlate with the age of onset of epilepsy, with the developmental delay usually becoming evident in infancy or childhood.[157]

Each of the DEEs with onset in childhood have variable ages of onset and are not self-limited (do not resolve). DEEs are characterized by developmental delay and may have other associated comorbidities. Seizures may be very difficult to control and may be drug resistant.

DEEs with onset in childhood include:

- Epilepsy with myoclonic-atonic seizures (previously known as Doose syndrome; also known as epilepsy with myoclonicastatic seizures)
- Lennox-Gastaut syndrome
- Landau Kleffner syndrome
- Developmental epileptic encephalopathy with continuous spike-wave activation in sleep (DEE-SWAS) and epileptic encephalopathy with spike-wave activation in sleep (EE-SWAS) (previously known as electrical status epilepticus in sleep, or ESES)

- Hemiconvulsion-hemiplegia-epilepsy syndrome
- Rasmussen syndrome

Three of the more common DEEs with onset in childhood are discussed below. Expanded information about the other syndromes with onset in childhood is available in Appendix 6 (online).

a) Epilepsy with myoclonic-atonic seizures

Epilepsy with myoclonic-atonic seizures (previously known as Doose syndrome; also known as epilepsy with myoclonic-astatic seizures) has an age of onset of between six months and six years and is often accompanied by developmental delays.[168] It is characterized by generalized tonic-clonic seizures, myoclonic seizures, myoclonic-atonic seizures, absence seizures, and status epilepticus. The onset of seizures is often abrupt.[168] A history of febrile seizures is present in one-fourth of cases, and a family history of seizures is present in one-third of cases.[168,169]

Comorbidities include intellectual disability, behavior disorders, sleep disorders, and movement disorders.[168] Often, comorbidities improve with seizure control. Management of epilepsy with myoclonic-atonic seizures involves antiseizure medications, although seizures are often drug resistant. The ketogenic diet may also be considered. Epilepsy resolves in two-thirds of cases.[168]

b) Lennox-Gastaut syndrome

Lennox-Gastaut syndrome has an age of onset of 18 months to 8 years.[168] Developmental delay is severe and may be present before the onset of seizures.[170] This syndrome is characterized by tonic or atonic seizures, or subtle absence seizures, although any seizure type can occur. About 30 percent of children with Lennox-Gastaut syndrome have a history of West syndrome.[171] Typically, Lennox-Gastaut syndrome occurs without any previous family history, and structural causes are common.[168]

Comorbidities include intellectual disability, behavior disorders, sleep disorders, and autism spectrum disorders.[172] Management is challenging and may include trying antiseizure medication such as cannabidiol (an antiseizure medication derived from the cannabis plant, known as medical cannabis), the ketogenic diet, neuromodulation, or epilepsy surgery.[161] In 80 to 90 percent of cases, seizures will continue into adulthood.[173]

c) Landau-Kleffner syndrome

Landau-Kleffner syndrome (considered a subtype of EE-SWAS) has an age of onset of between three and eight years.[174] It is characterized by a progressive loss of both speech and comprehension of speech. Obvious seizures occur in approximately 70 percent of individuals and often present as absence or focal seizures.[175] Speech delays and regression may persist in individuals even if seizures resolve.[176] The cause is genetic, although a family history is typically not present.[177]

Comorbidities include behavior disorders, ADHD (attention deficit hyperactivity disorder), cognitive impairment, depression, anxiety, and sleep disorders.[177] Management of Landau-Kleffner syndrome involves antiseizure medications, steroids, or epilepsy surgery.[174]

Generalized epilepsy syndromes

Generalized epilepsy syndromes with onset in childhood are genetic or *presumed* genetic and are characterized by generalized seizures. A family history may be present, and seizures may respond to antiseizure medications or may be drug resistant. The developmental impact ranges from unaffected to severe intellectual disability.

Generalized epilepsy syndromes with onset in childhood include:

- Childhood absence epilepsy (CAE)
- Epilepsy with myoclonic-absences
- Epilepsy with eyelid myoclonias (previously known as Jeavons syndrome)

CAE is one generalized epilepsy syndrome with onset in childhood and is described in detail below. Expanded information about the other generalized epilepsy syndromes with onset in childhood is available in Appendix 6 (online).

CAE has an age of onset of 2 to 12 years.[178] and is characterized by absence seizures that occur multiple times per day, lasting less than 20 seconds. These seizures may be provoked by hyperventilation. Developmental delays may occur.[179] A history of febrile seizures is present in 10 to 15 percent of cases, and about one-third of individuals with CAE have a family history of absence or other generalized seizures.[178,180]

Comorbidities include ADHD, learning disorders, behavior disorders, or psychiatric disorders, but overall development is typically normal.[179,181,182] Management of CAE involves antiseizure medications and, for many, seizures usually resolve by age 10 to 14.[179] Some will go on to develop juvenile absence epilepsy (JAE) or juvenile myoclonic epilepsy (JME).[178]

Note that CAE is also included within a group of epilepsy syndromes known as *genetic* generalized epilepsy (GGE, also known as idiopathic generalized epilepsy, or IGE). GGE/IGE also includes the following, which are addressed in section 7.4:

- Juvenile absence epilepsy (JAE)
- Juvenile myoclonic epilepsy (JME)
- Epilepsy with generalized tonic-clonic seizures alone

7.4 Onset in adolescence and adulthood

> As you grow older, you will discover that you have two hands,
> one for helping yourself, the other for helping others.
> **Audrey Hepburn**

Adolescence is the period between ages 10 and 19 years of age, and adulthood begins at 19 years of age.[49] Epilepsy syndromes in this age group include:

- Focal epilepsy syndromes
- Generalized epilepsy syndromes

Focal epilepsy syndromes

Focal epilepsy syndromes with onset in adolescence and adulthood are characterized by focal seizures that are often mild and infrequent. These syndromes are well controlled with antiseizure medications, and there is typically no developmental impact or associated comorbidities. Focal epilepsy syndromes with onset in adolescence and adulthood include:

- Autosomal dominant epilepsy with auditory features
- Other familial temporal lobe epilepsies

Generalized epilepsy syndromes

Generalized epilepsy syndromes with onset in adolescence and adulthood are characterized by generalized seizures that often require lifelong antiseizure medications to control.[183] These syndromes are genetic generalized epilepsy (GGE, also known as idiopathic generalized epilepsy or IGE) syndromes and are *presumed* to have a genetic cause, despite having no link to a specific gene.[181] Childhood absence epilepsy (described in the previous section) is also considered a genetic generalized epilepsy or an idiopathic generalized epilepsy). GGE/IGE often persists into adulthood and, as a group, accounts for 15 to 20 percent of all epilepsy cases in adults.[184] These syndromes may be accompanied by challenges with learning and attention, but development is typically normal. Generalized epilepsy syndromes with onset in adolescence and adulthood include:

- Juvenile absence epilepsy (JAE)
- Juvenile myoclonic epilepsy (JME)
- Epilepsy with generalized tonic-clonic seizures alone

Two of the more common generalized epilepsy syndromes with onset in adolescence and adulthood are JAE and JME, which are described below. Expanded information about the other syndromes with onset in adolescence and adulthood is available in Appendix 6 (online).

a) Juvenile absence epilepsy

Juvenile absence epilepsy (JAE) has an age of onset of between 8 and 20 years and is characterized by absence seizures as well as generalized tonic-clonic seizures and myoclonic jerks.[185,186] A family history of seizures or epilepsy is present in 42 percent of cases. In some individuals, JME may develop.[186]

b) Juvenile myoclonic epilepsy

Juvenile myoclonic epilepsy (JME) has an age of onset of 8 to 40 years and is characterized by myoclonic jerks, generalized tonic-clonic seizures, or absence seizures.[187] Seizures may be triggered by sleep deprivation, stress, or flashing light.[188] JME may evolve from CAE or JAE.[187]

7.5 Onset at a variable age

Life's most persistent and urgent question is, "What are you doing for others?"
Dr. Martin Luther King Jr.

Some epilepsy syndromes may occasionally occur at a different age than what is listed above, and theoretically they could be included in this section. However, some epilepsy syndromes are *known* to occur at variable ages.

Epilepsy syndromes with onset at a variable age include:

- Reflex epilepsy (reading epilepsy and startle epilepsy)
- Familial focal epilepsy with variable foci
- Progressive myoclonus epilepsies
- Sleep-related hypermotor (hyperkinetic) epilepsy (SHE, previously known as nocturnal frontal lobe epilepsy)
- Mesial temporal lobe epilepsy with hippocampal sclerosis (MTLE-HS)
- Febrile infection related epilepsy syndrome (FIRES)

Reading epilepsy (a type of reflex epilepsy) is one epilepsy syndrome with onset at a variable age and is described below. Expanded information about the other syndromes with onset at a variable age is available in Appendix 6 (online).

Reading epilepsy is associated with reflex seizures that occur after a particular stimulus (i.e., reading). Reading epilepsy (also termed "epilepsy with reading-induced seizures") has an age of onset of between 12 and 19 years and is characterized by myoclonic jerks and generalized tonic-clonic seizures, which are triggered in response to reading. Individuals diagnosed with reading epilepsy may have a family history of epilepsy (20 to 40 percent).[189] Development is typically normal, and usually there are no associated comorbidities. Management of reading epilepsy is with antiseizure medications and by limiting reading.

Key points Chapter 7

- An epilepsy syndrome is a group of symptoms consistently occurring together, associated with the diagnosis of epilepsy.
- Identifying the epilepsy syndrome can often be more important than identifying the cause of epilepsy for deciding management, which makes this step of the diagnostic journey very important.
- The identification of an epilepsy syndrome is more common when the onset of epilepsy is in the neonatal period, infancy, or childhood compared with onset in adulthood.
- Epilepsy syndromes may be identified by characteristics including the age of epilepsy onset, seizure type, cause, and developmental impact.
- Many epilepsy syndromes have a developmental impact that results in a delay in meeting developmental milestones.
- Epilepsy syndromes with onset in the neonatal period and infancy include self-limited epilepsy syndromes, developmental and epileptic encephalopathies, and etiology-specific syndromes.
- Epilepsy syndromes with onset in childhood include self-limited focal epilepsy syndromes, developmental and epileptic encephalopathies, and generalized epilepsy syndromes.
- Epilepsy syndromes with onset in adolescence and adulthood include focal epilepsy syndromes and generalized epilepsy syndromes.
- Other epilepsy syndromes may have an onset at a variable age.

Chapter 8

Management of epilepsy

Section 8.1 Introduction 163
Section 8.2 Pharmaceutical management 168
Section 8.3 Non-pharmaceutical management 182
Section 8.4 Other medications or supplements 199
Section 8.5 Alternative and complementary therapies 205
Key points Chapter 8 209

8.1 Introduction

If you treat an individual as he is, he will remain how he is. But if you treat him as if he were what he ought to be and could be, he will become what he ought to be and could be.

Johann Wolfgang von Goethe

The difference in meaning between "management" and "treatment" is subtle. "Management" is the broader term, considering all aspects of an individual's life, whereas "treatment" is the use of a specific intervention, such as medication or surgery. Management and treatment aim to promote optimal participation in daily life by enhancing activities and minimizing problems with body functions and structure. Varying treatment options are available for epilepsy, but all need to be considered under the broad topic of management, ensuring all aspects of the individual's life are considered. Therefore, the term "management" is used here when referring to both the overall management and the individual treatments used for epilepsy.

The management of epilepsy generally includes:

- **Pharmaceutical management,** involving the use of antiseizure medications, as monotherapy or polytherapy
- **Non-pharmaceutical management,** involving the ketogenic diet, neuromodulation (repetitive electrical discharges administered through a surgically implanted device), and epilepsy surgery
- **Other medications or supplements,** including vitamins or medical cannabis

Pharmaceutical treatments are generally tried first. However, some epilepsy syndromes and drug-resistant epilepsy are best managed with non-pharmaceutical treatments or other medications or supplements. Pharmaceutical, non-pharmaceutical, and other medications or supplements can be used with the same individual and at the same time. With any treatment, long-term monitoring is required while treatment is ongoing.

Goals of epilepsy management

Recall from section 2.6 that one of the main goals of epilepsy management is to *prevent, reduce,* or *stop* seizures. Central to epilepsy management are the concepts of seizure control and seizure freedom, both of which may be achieved through effective epilepsy management.

- **Seizure control** refers to a decrease in frequency, severity, and/or duration of seizures.
- **Seizure freedom** is a set period of time without any seizures. It is the ultimate goal, although achieving this is not possible for every individual.

To determine seizure freedom, the ILAE suggests using a rule of three: a length of time that is three times longer than the longest length of time between seizures in an individual before starting treatment. For example, if an individual previously had seizures every one to three months, a period of nine months without seizures would need to pass (3 x 3 = 9) before they could be classed as seizure-free. Alternatively, a period of 12 months without any seizures may be used.

Effective epilepsy management, which achieves seizure control or seizure freedom, prevents individuals from experiencing breakthrough seizures, seizure clusters, or status epilepticus.

- **Breakthrough seizures** are those that occur despite the individual taking ongoing (at least daily) antiseizure medication.
- **Seizure clusters** are repetitive seizures (more than two in 24 hours) occurring despite the individual taking ongoing antiseizure medications.
- **Status epilepticus,** a life-threatening condition, is defined as seizures lasting more than five minutes, or multiple generalized onset seizures occurring in close succession (one after the other, without a return to baseline).[2]

Why manage epilepsy?

Management of epilepsy is important to:

- Protect the brain from damage
- Protect organs and body systems from damage
- Prevent status epilepticus
- Prevent sudden unexpected death in epilepsy (SUDEP)
- Ensure safety and prevent injury
- Improve quality of life

a) Protect the brain from damage

Damage from epileptic seizures may include the loss of neurons, changes in the structure of the brain, or changes in function. This is particularly relevant when drug-resistant epilepsy occurs. Children with drug-resistant epilepsy are at risk of cognitive, behavioral, and psychiatric conditions.[32]

b) Protect organs and body systems from damage

Epileptic seizures (especially those with motor signs) may lead to injuries and lesions in various body organs (i.e., kidneys or liver), or body systems (i.e., cardiovascular system or musculoskeletal system).

In turn, such injuries and lesions may lead to long-term consequences (including SUDEP).

c) Prevent status epilepticus

Status epilepticus markedly increases the risk of brain damage and may lead to death.[190]

d) Prevent SUDEP

SUDEP is a rare complication of epilepsy—the unexpected death of an individual with epilepsy when no other cause of death can be found.

e) Ensure safety and prevent injury

Even when seizures are controlled, individuals with epilepsy are at a higher risk of injury than the general population from falls, motor vehicle accidents, and accidents around water, fire, and other activities. The risk is most pronounced in the first two years following seizure onset.[32,191] Individuals with drug-resistant epilepsy and those with comorbidities are at a higher risk of seizure-related injuries.[32,191] Education related to preventive and safety measures is a key part of overall epilepsy management.

f) Improve quality of life

The unpredictable nature of seizures and the lack of control may have a negative impact on the quality of life of individuals with epilepsy.[192] Seizure control correlates with the ability to participate fully in life, including social activities, physical activities, education, employment, driving, and independent living. Misunderstandings about epilepsy can be found throughout history and still exist in many cultures around the world.[134] These can lead to undue restrictions for individuals with epilepsy.

Prognosis

"Prognosis" means the "prospect of recovering from injury or disease, or a prediction or forecast of the course and outcome of a medical condition."[193] For some individuals, epilepsy is a lifelong chronic condition,* while for many others, the prognosis with epilepsy is good and the condition resolves.[194,195]

Key terms related to epilepsy prognosis include:

- **Remission:** A state where an individual with epilepsy is seizure-free for at least six months. Remission criteria vary, however, and for some individuals, a longer time period may be used (such as two years or five years).
- **Resolved:** A state where an individual with epilepsy has remained seizure-free for the last 10 years, with no antiseizure medications for the last 5 years, or where the individual had an age-dependent epilepsy syndrome and is now past the applicable age for this diagnosis (i.e., self-limited neonatal or infantile epilepsy syndromes).[5]

Research shows:

- Epilepsy in children often resolves, and about 60 percent of those with childhood-onset epilepsy achieve a five-year remission period and can stop antiseizure medication.[66]
- In individuals of all ages with epilepsy, 64 percent taking antiseizure medication experience 12 months or more of seizure freedom and 55 to 68 percent experience prolonged seizure remission.[66,196]
- In those with prolonged seizure remission, about half will remain seizure-free after discontinuing antiseizure medication.[197]

Some indicators correlate with better epilepsy prognosis. These include:[66]

- Early response to treatment such as a positive response to the first two antiseizure medications in the first two years of treatment
- Lower number of seizures at the time of diagnosis of epilepsy
- Epilepsy with a certain genetic or presumed genetic cause (compared to epilepsy with a structural or metabolic cause)
- No history of generalized tonic-clonic seizures

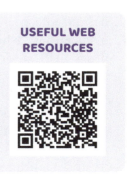

USEFUL WEB RESOURCES

---

* A condition lasting more than one year and requiring ongoing medical attention and/or causing the individual to limit some activities of daily living.

8.2

Pharmaceutical management

> A plan is what, a schedule is when.
> It takes both a plan and a schedule
> to get things done.
> **Peter Turla**

The pharmaceutical management of epilepsy is complex and aims to *prevent, reduce,* or *stop* seizures while minimizing the risk of adverse side effects from medication. (Adverse side effects are unintended and potentially harmful outcomes that occur in addition to a treatment's desired effect.) Pharmaceutical management is done with antiseizure medications, which are also known as anticonvulsants, antiepileptic drugs (AEDs), or simply seizure medications or seizure drugs.

Parents of young children and individuals with epilepsy should have a good understanding of the principles of antiseizure medications. Medical professionals will guide the specific medication choices, but parents (and individuals with epilepsy) will have the bulk of the responsibility for medication management—deciding to give rescue medication, monitoring for behavioral changes, managing their child when sick, alerting others who interact with their child about potential adverse side effects, and sticking to a strict medication schedule. Understanding these principles is more important than knowing specific details of each antiseizure medication.

Pharmaceutical management with antiseizure medications involves understanding:

- **Monotherapy versus polytherapy**
- **The history of antiseizure medication development**
- **Ongoing antiseizure medication versus seizure rescue medication**
- **Principles of medication management: Important considerations**
- **Levels of pharmaceutical management**
- **Factors affecting antiseizure medication choice**
- **Mechanism of action**
- **Adverse side effects**
- **Illness and antiseizure medication**

a) Monotherapy versus polytherapy

Often, the first step in epilepsy management is starting one antiseizure medication, which is known as monotherapy ("mono" means one).[198] It is important that sufficient time be given to try the antiseizure medication as the effectiveness may not be immediately apparent. "Sufficient time" can be weeks or even months; patience is required to find the right medication for the individual. If one single antiseizure medication doesn't work, a different single one might be tried.

If different single medications are not effective, more than one antiseizure medication may be used together, which is known as polytherapy ("poly" means many).[199] Varying combinations of antiseizure medications may be tried. If the seizures stop (with either monotherapy or polytherapy) and seizure freedom is achieved, the epilepsy may be described as being "drug responsive."[200]

When two appropriately used antiseizure medications (used together, in polytherapy) fail to achieve seizure freedom, the epilepsy may be described as "drug resistant" (also referred to as drug-refractory, pharmacoresistant, or uncontrolled epilepsy).[201] This does not mean, however, that additional antiseizure medications will fail to achieve seizure freedom; for some individuals, more than two antiseizure medications may be recommended. Individuals with drug-resistant epilepsy may still use antiseizure medications to help decrease the frequency, duration, or severity of seizures, even if the medications do not completely stop them. In addition, non-pharmaceutical management may be indicated for drug-resistant epilepsy (see section 8.3).

While everyone responds differently to antiseizure medications, studies have shown:

- For 47 percent of individuals with epilepsy, monotherapy with a first antiseizure medication results in seizure freedom, and for 13 percent, monotherapy with a second antiseizure medication results in seizure freedom.[202]
- For approximately 20 to 25 percent of children and one-third of adults with epilepsy, antiseizure medication alone is not enough to provide seizure freedom, and drug-resistant epilepsy is diagnosed, which requires further interventions.[201]
- The World Health Organization estimates around 70 percent of people living with epilepsy could be seizure-free with appropriate antiseizure medications.[21,24]

Although antiseizure medications may work to effectively control seizures in most people with epilepsy, adverse side effects may be experienced.

A link to a comprehensive list of antiseizure medications can be found in **Useful web resources**.

b) The history of antiseizure medication development

Antiseizure medications are continually being developed, and it is not possible to cover all antiseizure medications in this book. Included in this chapter are names of some common antiseizure medications, but note that not all medications are available in all countries, and some may be known by different names. In addition, certain medications are approved by some health care and insurance systems, while others are not. Some health systems may require an individual to try certain medications before moving onto others. Questions about specific medications should always be directed to a medical professional.

Figure 8.2.1 (on the next page) is a timeline of antiseizure medication development beginning in the 1800s. The medications (drugs) are classified as first-, second-, or third-generation, denoting the time when they were introduced. Some first-generation medications are still in use today, have been well studied, and may be very effective. First-generation medications may require additional laboratory testing (e.g., kidney and liver function), are often not appropriate to take during pregnancy, and may have more adverse side effects compared with newer (second- or third-generation) antiseizure medications. Second- and third-generation antiseizure medications are less likely to cause drug–drug interactions, are associated with fewer adverse side effects (requiring less laboratory testing), and may be safer to take during pregnancy when compared to first-generation antiseizure medications. However, newer antiseizure medications are more expensive and may be more difficult to obtain (particularly third-generation medications).

Despite the advances and increase in available antiseizure medications, the rates of drug-resistant epilepsy have not changed much since the introduction of the first-generation medications.[198] A link to a comprehensive list of antiseizure medications can be found in **Useful web resources**.

c) Ongoing antiseizure medication versus seizure rescue medication

In general, antiseizure medications are either ongoing or seizure rescue medications. Each has its own use, and each is administered differently:

- **Ongoing antiseizure medications** are administered daily or multiple times per day. They are sometimes referred to as chronic antiseizure medications. The most common routes for administering them are oral (by mouth) and enteral (G-tubes or J-tubes*).
- **Seizure rescue medications** are administered only during active seizures. The oral or enteral routes are not typically a safe and appropriate option, so seizure rescue medications are typically given through an alternate route, including:

---

* Gastrostomy and jejunostomy tubes (G-tubes and J-tubes) are inserted through a surgical opening in the stomach or small intestine and provide an alternate route for nutrition, fluids, or medications.

- Rectal (in a liquid or gel form inserted into the rectum)
- Intranasal (in a spray form, into the nostrils)
- Buccal (between the gums and the cheeks allowing absorption by the mucous membranes in the mouth)
- When available, intravenous (IV) or intramuscular (IM)

Seizure rescue medications are generally from a class of medications known as benzodiazepines, such as diazepam, midazolam, and lorazepam. Benzodiazepines act quickly to depress or sedate the central nervous system, which includes lowering breathing and heart rate, and inducing drowsiness. After administering seizure rescue medication, it is important to monitor the individual for adverse side effects (e.g., problems with breathing, oversedation).[203]

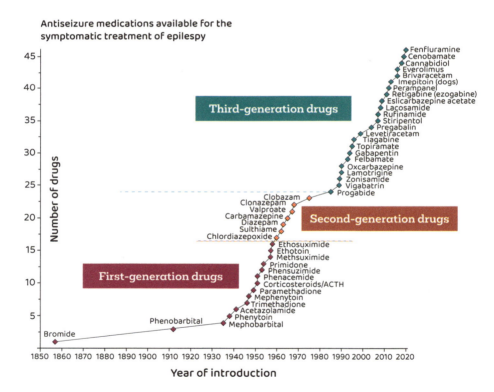

Figure 8.2.1 Timeline of antiseizure medication development. Adapted from "The Pharmacology and Clinical Efficacy of Antiseizure Medications: From bromide salts to cenobamate and beyond," by W. Loscher and P. Klein (2021). Used under a Creative Commons Attribution-Noncommercial 4.0 International License. https://creativecommons.org/licenses/by-nc/4.0/

Seizure rescue medications are recommended for any seizure that lasts more than three to five minutes. The timing of administering the medication is important because it may take two to three minutes for it to take effect. Usually, seizures will stop by themselves in under five minutes, but seizures that last more than five minutes are likely to continue even longer, which may increase the risk of long-term neurological effects like brain damage.

d) Principles of medication management: Important considerations

With any medication, how it is administered, monitored, and managed is crucial to its effectiveness. Parents of children and adolescents with epilepsy, and the individuals themselves when they are old enough, should understand the following principles and terms used with medication administration.

i) Ongoing antiseizure medications

- **Dosage:** The full prescribed dose should always be administered. Underdosing will not be effective. Antiseizure medications, particularly in infants and children, are dosed based on the weight of the individual. As the child grows and gains weight, the dose may need to be adjusted.
- **Timing:** Antiseizure medications should ideally be taken as close as possible to the same time each day (e.g., every 12 hours or every 24 hours). This is a general rule and will vary on the specific antiseizure medication, so consulting with the medical professional is important. Many medications have a narrow therapeutic range, meaning that there is a small margin between the effective dosage and the dosage that can cause damage (toxicity) to the body, resulting in adverse side effects. It's important to avoid missing a dose of ongoing antiseizure medication, as the risk of breakthrough seizures will increase. The most common cause of breakthrough seizures is noncompliance with antiseizure medication. (Breakthrough seizures are those that occur in an individual with epilepsy despite ongoing antiseizure medication.)
- **Titration:** Titration is the process of slowly adjusting medication dosages to achieve optimal effects while minimizing adverse side effects. Antiseizure medications are prescribed at low doses to start

and are gradually increased over time. Since the same dose does not work for everyone, starting with a low dose, allowing the medication to build up in the blood, and monitoring for therapeutic levels (see below) and adverse side effects are recommended.[204] This can take days to weeks.

- **Therapeutic level:** "Therapeutic level" refers to the specific concentration of an antiseizure medication in the blood that is effective for controlling seizures in an individual. "Therapeutic range" describes the lower and upper concentration within which the medication is considered effective for controlling seizures but is not toxic. Therapeutic monitoring measures the concentration of medication within the blood at specific intervals of time, since it changes depending on when the last medication dose is taken. The concentration measured immediately before the first dose of medication in the morning is known as a trough level, which is the lowest amount of the medication in the blood before the next dose. Depending on the results of the therapeutic monitoring, the dose may need to be adjusted. Doses that are too low may not be effective, and doses that are too high may cause damage (toxicity) to the body and may result in adverse side effects.
- **Long-term monitoring:** It's important that long-term monitoring be carried out for anyone taking ongoing antiseizure medications. This is done with regular blood tests. A complete blood count measures the levels of blood components, including red blood cells, white blood cells, hemoglobin, hematocrit, and platelets. Other lab tests evaluate the function of the kidneys, liver, and levels of vitamins and minerals. The frequency of these tests will vary depending on the specific antiseizure medication and comorbidities.
- **Medication interaction:** All medications have the potential to interact with other medications. Parents of children with epilepsy, or the individual themselves, should tell the medical professional about *all* medications being taken, including those not related to epilepsy, and any nonprescription drugs (e.g., ibuprofen).
- **Weaning:** When an antiseizure medication needs to be stopped, it typically needs to be done gradually, with the dose decreased over time, in a process known as weaning. Weaning schedules should be carefully followed to prevent seizures that can occur when antiseizure medications are withdrawn too quickly. This can take weeks to months.

- **Adjustments for travel:** When crossing time zones, medication timing should be adjusted as needed. For short trips that cross only a few time zones, the medication can be taken at the "new" time (e.g., if medication is normally taken at 9 a.m. on Pacific time, it should be taken at noon on Eastern time). For longer trips or when crossing several time zones, the timing should be adjusted gradually (e.g., if crossing eight time zones ahead, the medication should be taken 30 to 60 minutes later than usual on the old time until the time has "caught up" to the new time zone). Individuals should identify a pharmacy close to their destination and discuss alternate plans for medications, if needed, with their medical professional before travel.

ii) Seizure rescue medications

- **Dosage:** The full prescribed dose should always be administered. Underdosing will not be effective. It is important when administering seizure rescue medication that the person administering it does *not* just give a small amount in hopes the seizure will stop.
- **Expiration and refills:** Since seizure rescue medications are typically not used often, the expiration date should be noted so that refills are arranged before that date. The medications are typically prescribed in a single-dose format, so once the medication is used, it will have to be refilled for future use.
- **Keep medication with the individual:** Anywhere the individual goes, the seizure rescue medication should go. This includes daycare, school, work, and other events. Anyone supervising an individual with epilepsy should know how and when to administer the seizure rescue medication.
- **Route of medication delivery:** In school or other public settings, the rectal route for seizure rescue medication is not the best choice—the intranasal or buccal routes are preferred. If the individual has a severe runny nose or severe nasal congestion, the intranasal may not be the best route. In that case, the rectal or buccal routes might be better. Also, if there are anal or rectal problems (e.g., anal fissures—small tears or cracks in the anus), it might be best to avoid the rectal route and use the nasal or buccal route instead.
- **Adjustments for travel:** Having enough medication on hand for travel must also be considered. But note that some countries may restrict bringing in seizure rescue medications, so it's important to

check before travel. As well, individuals should identify a pharmacy close to their destination and discuss alternate plans for medications, if needed, with their medical professional before travel.

e) Levels of pharmaceutical management

In general, the levels of pharmaceutical management move from the least intensive or aggressive (for epilepsy generally) to the most intensive (for status epilepticus). Each level describes the management needed for an individual with epilepsy at any given time.

- **Epilepsy:** The main goal is to prevent, reduce, or stop epileptic seizures with ongoing antiseizure medications. Individuals diagnosed with epilepsy will most often need these medications daily or multiple times per day.
- **Breakthrough seizures:** The main goal is to stop an active seizure that lasts for more than three to five minutes with seizure rescue medications. If breakthrough seizures occur, adjustments to the ongoing medications (either the dose or the medication itself) may be needed.
- **Seizure cluster:** The main goal is to stop seizure clusters with seizure rescue medications. Seizure clusters are concerning when they last longer or occur closer together as they may increase the risk of status epilepticus.[205]
- **Status epilepticus:** The main goal is to stop the ongoing persistent seizures occurring in close succession (one after the other, without a return to baseline) or seizures occurring continuously. Status epilepticus requires hospitalization and close monitoring along with seizure rescue medications. Ongoing EEG monitoring is also typically needed.

Figure 8.2.2 depicts the levels of pharmaceutical management in epilepsy.

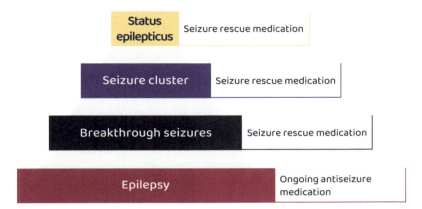

Figure 8.2.2 Levels of pharmaceutical management.[198] Adapted with kind permission from Dr. Anteneh M. Feyissa.

f) Factors affecting antiseizure medication choice

The choice of specific antiseizure medication is made after considering several factors. These factors vary by individual and include the type of seizure, type of epilepsy, epilepsy cause, epilepsy syndrome, sex, age, and comorbidities.

- **Type of seizure:** Some antiseizure medications should not be used for certain types of seizures. For example, some may worsen generalized seizures. One categorization of antiseizure medications is based on the therapeutic spectrum of the type of seizures they treat:
  - **Broad therapeutic spectrum**: These antiseizure medications impact a broad range of seizure types (both focal and generalized). When the seizure type is unknown, broad spectrum antiseizure medications are generally administered. Examples include clobazam, levetiracetam, lamotrigine, valproate, and topiramate.
  - **Narrow therapeutic spectrum**: These antiseizure medications work by targeting specific seizure types, like focal or absence seizures. Examples include carbamazepine, oxcarbazepine, and ethosuximide (absence seizures).
- **Type of epilepsy:** Some antiseizure medications are contraindicated for certain types of epilepsy, while others may be preferred for a particular epilepsy type.

- **Epilepsy cause:** Depending on the cause, some types of epilepsy are best treated with a combination of pharmaceutical and non-pharmaceutical treatments.
- **Epilepsy syndrome:** Some epilepsy syndromes respond well to specific antiseizure medications while others may be more responsive to other medications such as high-dose steroids or vitamin supplements.
- **Sex:** Biological sex is an important consideration when determining which antiseizure medication to administer.[206] Females may experience an increase in seizures related to their menstrual cycle (known as catamenial epilepsy), and adjustments to antiseizure medications may be needed during menstrual cycles. As well, a decrease in the effectiveness of hormonal birth control occurs with some antiseizure medications. (Considerations related to antiseizure medications and pregnancy are also important and are addressed in Chapter 10.)
- **Age:** Some medications are better suited for adults and may not be recommended for infants and children, and vice versa. Dosing considerations are typically based on the size of the individual, which often correlates with age.
- **Comorbidities:** Antiseizure medications may need to be adjusted based on comorbidities. Some are preferred with specific comorbidities, while others should be avoided or used with caution.

Note: Regulatory approvals vary by country, and antiseizure medication choice may be impacted by health care and insurance systems.

g) Mechanism of action

The mechanism of action of a medication refers to how a medication works in the body to achieve a desired effect. As it relates to antiseizure medications, it is what the medication does to prevent, reduce, or stop seizures. Even among experts, the precise mechanism of action of some antiseizure medications is not clear.

The mechanism of action of antiseizure medications typically occurs at the synapse—the space between neurons or between neurons and other cells. Antiseizure medications regulate how electrical activity moves through neurons and across synapses by influencing both ion flow and neurotransmitter activity. Specifically, they control the movement of ions such as sodium, potassium, and calcium through ion channels, and they regulate neurotransmitters that carry signals between neurons and other cells. By working at these levels, antiseizure medications help prevent the abnormal electrical activity that leads to seizures.

More information on the mechanism of action of antiseizure medications is included in Appendix 7 (online).

h) Adverse side effects

Antiseizure medications may cause adverse side effects, although these often improve over time or may be managed by adjusting the dose of the medication.

Almost always, the benefits of controlling the seizures with antiseizure medications should outweigh the adverse side effects. Any changes to antiseizure medications (especially the decision to discontinue taking them) need to be discussed with the medical professional.

If the dosage is outside the therapeutic range (too high, leading to toxicity), it may contribute to adverse side effects. Some investigations (i.e., genetic testing) might be helpful in assessing the risk of adverse side effects of certain antiseizure medications.*[207] Once the antiseizure medication is discontinued, adverse side effects usually resolve.

Common adverse side effects of antiseizure medications include dizziness, sleepiness, upset stomach, nausea, and constipation.[208–210]

Antiseizure medications may also lead to long-term side effects and contribute to the development of comorbidities. In some individuals, these are more challenging than the seizures themselves and are a common reason for people to change or stop antiseizure medications. Several studies address long-term side effects and comorbidities associated with antiseizure medication:

- Cognitive and behavioral changes and regression in developmental milestones may be due in part to antiseizure medication in children and are more severe with polytherapy.[211]

---

* One example of genetic testing related to antiseizure medication side effects is screening for the HLA-B*1502 allele (a particular variant of a gene), which is recommended prior to starting carbamazepine in individuals with Asian ancestry due to the risk of Stevens-Johnson syndrome and a severe adverse reaction known as toxic epidermal necrolysis.

- Antiseizure medications may result in attention disruptions and memory problems negatively impacting learning.[212,213] Cognitive slowing, or a decrease in mental processing speed, is a frequent complaint in individuals who are taking antiseizure medications.[213]
- Children who take antiseizure medication have increased rates of negative behavioral and emotional problems, especially when they take more than one (polytherapy).[103,211] Eleven percent of those age 2 to 18 years with epilepsy report either decreasing or discontinuing antiseizure medications due to psychiatric and behavioral adverse side effects.[214]
- Irritability and aggression occur in 10 to 16 percent of individuals with epilepsy taking antiseizure medication.[182]
- Antiseizure medications can exacerbate psychiatric symptoms and may increase thoughts of suicide.[215,216]
- Antiseizure medications may impair how vitamin D (important for bone health) is processed in the body and may contribute to the development of musculoskeletal comorbidities.[217,218]
- Cardiac arrythmias (atypical heart rhythms that may be too slow, too fast, or irregular) might develop with some antiseizure medications.[219,220]
- Some antiseizure medications are associated with increased rates of obesity, and others may be associated with weight loss.[221]
- Some antiseizure medications may contribute to bed-wetting (enuresis).[222] However, urinary incontinence due to nighttime seizures should be excluded before attributing the bed-wetting to a medication side effect.

Serious, life-threatening adverse side effects of antiseizure medications are also possible and require immediate medical attention. These include:

- Suicidal ideation[216]
- Stevens-Johnson syndrome (a severe disorder of the skin and mucous membranes resulting in a widespread rash)[223]

i) Illness and epilepsy management

Individuals with epilepsy experience typical illnesses like colds, influenza, and other viruses. These illnesses may trigger seizures and can also lead to missed doses of antiseizure medications, which may lead to breakthrough seizures.

General guidelines for managing epilepsy during illness include:

- Continue to take antiseizure medications on the scheduled timeline, whenever possible. This may require using an alternate route (e.g., using rectal instead of oral route when vomiting occurs, or having a medical professional administer the medication using intramuscular or intravenous route).
- Stay as hydrated as possible.
- Consult a medical professional before administering any other medications; even those obtained without a prescription, as some may interact with antiseizure medications.
- Follow the directions and dosages for seizure rescue medications if needed.

8.3 Non-pharmaceutical management

> You don't have to see the whole staircase,
> just take the first step.
> **Dr. Martin Luther King Jr.**

When antiseizure medications fail to provide seizure freedom, non-pharmaceutical management may be considered. Non-pharmaceutical management is often used alongside antiseizure medications for those who have drug-resistant epilepsy. Some types of epilepsy and some epilepsy syndromes respond better to non-pharmaceutical management, and in these cases, it may be used instead of antiseizure medications. Non-pharmaceutical management includes:

- **The ketogenic diet**
- **Neuromodulation**
- **Epilepsy surgery**

The ketogenic diet

The ketogenic diet is a form of dietary therapy that restricts the intake of carbohydrates, allows for a moderate amount of protein, and greatly increases the intake of fats to induce a metabolic state known as ketosis. In ketosis, the body and brain use fats (released as ketones) instead of glucose (from carbohydrates) for energy.[224]

The exact mechanism by which ketosis works to control seizures is not fully understood, but it is thought to decrease neuron excitability and increase inhibitory neurotransmitters, both which work to control seizures.[225] Recall from section 3.3. that neurotransmitters act in the area of the synapse to either excite the next neuron or cell, or inhibit the next neuron or cell. Despite the diet's potential benefit, for most individuals, antiseizure medications are typically taken along with the ketogenic diet for the management of epilepsy.

Note that the ketogenic diet for epilepsy is much more rigid than the "keto" diet that has gained popularity for weight loss. The ketogenic diet is not something an individual can or should start and stop like other diets. "Cheat meals" or other variations to the diet are not allowed. The ketogenic diet should be thought of as a medication needed consistently, without missing any doses. Consultation with a dietitian is essential.

Variations of the ketogenic diet do exist, but the most common one used for epilepsy is the "classic ketogenic diet," which has been around for over a century. The ketogenic diet is prescribed for each individual as a specific daily total number of calories to be consumed as a ratio of grams of fats to grams of protein and carbohydrates combined. The best ratio for each individual depends on the optimum seizure control needed, compliance ability, and side effects. The ketogenic diet ratio most recommended for children with epilepsy is 4:1 or 3:1. (A 3:1 ratio may be used when compliance with the 4:1 ratio is poor.)

Figure 8.3.1 shows a typical breakdown of fats, carbohydrates, and protein in the ketogenic diet with a ratio of 4:1—that is, the calories from fat are four times the calories from carbohydrates and proteins combined. In the 4:1 ratio, 90 percent of the calories come from fats.[226]

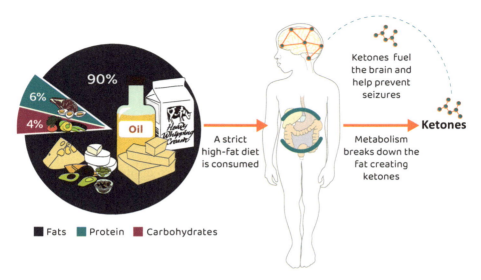

Figure 8.3.1 Ketogenic diet calorie distribution in a 4:1 ratio.

The fats prescribed typically include butter, oils, mayonnaise, and heavy whipping cream in addition to fats from nuts, avocado, and cheeses. Anything the individual takes in by mouth must be measured and tracked, including nonfoods such as toothpaste and mouthwash, chewable or liquid medications, vitamins, and chewing gum, all of which may contain carbohydrates. The full amount of calories from fats, carbohydrates, and protein in the prescribed ratio needs to be consumed each day.

Following a ketogenic diet is a big commitment. In addition to weighing and measuring food, families may need to learn to monitor ketone levels at home with a ketone meter (or for adolescents and adults, they need to do this themselves). The use of a ketone meter should be coordinated with the medical professional. Regular follow-up appointments are needed, typically at least every three months.

The ketogenic diet is often initiated during a hospital stay where the individual can be monitored for seizures and treated for adverse side effects (see below). Because the diet is associated with adverse side effects in individuals of all ages, initiating it at home requires keeping close contact with medical professionals.

Following are notes on monitoring and managing the adverse side effects of the ketogenic diet that may occur:

- Sleepiness and fatigue are common side effects, especially at the beginning of the diet, though this usually improves with time.
- Gastrointestinal issues such as vomiting, diarrhea, and constipation occur in 30 percent and are typically managed with medications or adjustments to the diet.[227]
- Slow and reduced growth and decreased weight gain affects growing children.[228] Monitoring weight and height frequently is recommended.[229,230] A specific test, known as a bone age test (an X-ray), may be used to evaluate the growth of the child.
- Levels of vitamin D and calcium may be decreased, which may lead to fractures.[229] Laboratory testing of levels in the blood is recommended; vitamin and mineral supplements are needed while on the diet.[228]
- Changes in the blood levels of certain nutrients and elements may occur, including low blood glucose levels (hypoglycemia), electrolyte changes, deficiencies in some elements (e.g., carnitine, which helps with energy metabolism), and increased levels of lipids (high cholesterol).[231] Frequent monitoring with laboratory tests is recommended as well as ECG monitoring for any cardiac arrythmias due to electrolyte changes. A glucometer may be used at home to monitor blood glucose levels. A small amount of sugar may be administered if indicated.
- Dehydration may occur, and keeping well hydrated is particularly important. Checking the specific gravity of the urine* and monitoring for appropriate output of urine is required.
- Kidney stones may occur in about 3 to 7 percent of children who are on the diet. Monitoring for kidney stones with renal ultrasound may be recommended.[229]

Because staying on the ketogenic diet requires much effort, compliance is a primary influence on its effectiveness. For infants and children, the effort and compliance must come from the parents, and require commitment and acceptance that the stress of maintaining this diet may actually increase over time.[230] Infants and children who are tube-fed

---

* Specific gravity is a measure of the concentration of urine. Abnormal results may indicate dehydration or kidney abnormalities.

have high levels of compliance following a ketogenic diet, while adolescents and older children (who eat orally) may not cooperate with it.[232] Overall compliance with a classic ketogenic diet in adults is only around 38 percent.[233]

Compliance can be particularly challenging when individuals with epilepsy experience typical illnesses like colds, influenza, and other viruses. Being ill may make it more likely that the ketogenic diet is disrupted. The medical professional can provide specific sick day guidelines for a ketogenic diet, which should be followed carefully.

In terms of effectiveness of the ketogenic diet, it has been reported that:

- When the diet is followed, it may result in good seizure control (a decrease in the frequency, severity, and/or duration of seizures).[227] These effects may be noted immediately or may take one to three months. An added benefit is higher rates of productivity, reduced anxiety, and better cognitive functioning.[227]
- In children age 2 to 16 years with epilepsy, 38 percent experienced a greater than 50 percent reduction in seizures after three months of following the diet.[234]
- Up to 10 to 15 percent of children may become seizure-free on the diet while also continuing antiseizure medications, and sometimes with fewer medications or smaller doses.[235]
- Children with certain types of epilepsy and epilepsy syndromes, such as Lennox-Gastaut, West, Dravet, GLUT1 deficiency, and others may particularly benefit from the ketogenic diet.[224]

If seizures are well controlled and the ketogenic diet is tolerated, individuals may remain on it for two years. After that time, the diet is gradually stopped (over several months) and the individual returns to a regular diet. Generally, individuals cannot remain on the ketogenic diet long-term due to its side effects, such as increased cholesterol, which can lead to cardiovascular issues. In certain circumstances, the ketogenic diet is used long-term: when it's the only effective treatment for controlling seizures or when the seizures are due to metabolic causes or epilepsy syndromes, such as GLUT1 deficiency syndrome.

Finding support groups and outlets to manage the stress associated with following this diet is important. Websites for helpful organizations are included in **Useful web resources**.

Neuromodulation

Neuromodulation is the alteration (modulation) of neurons (neuro) and their communication networks by using targeted electrical stimulation.[236] When used in the management of epilepsy, it involves the surgical implantation of a medical device (neuromodulation device) that administers repetitive electrical discharges to disrupt the neuron communication networks that cause seizures in order to reduce, prevent, or stop the seizures.

Different therapeutic neuromodulation devices are used in the management of epilepsy including:

- **Vagus nerve stimulation (VNS)**
- **Responsive neurostimulation (RNS)**
- **Deep brain stimulation (DBS)**

Neuromodulation devices may be sensitive to electromagnetic fields such as those in MRI, metal detectors, or large electronic devices. Once a neuromodulation device is implanted, the individual receives a special ID card with information about the device and instructions for safety related to electromagnetic fields.

a) Vagus nerve stimulation

The vagus nerve stimulation (VNS) device is surgically implanted and programmed to periodically stimulate the vagus nerve, which is a cranial nerve that affects multiple areas in the body, including the throat, tongue, lungs, heart, and digestive system.[237] Stimulation of the vagus nerve has been shown to stop seizure activity.

The VNS device is implanted under the skin, in the left upper chest area, and the wires (also known as leads) attached to the device are placed near the left vagus nerve[199] (see Figure 8.3.2). The VNS device works by sending regular, mild pulses of electrical energy to the brain via the vagus nerve.[238] The pulses are mild and the individual cannot usually feel them.[238]

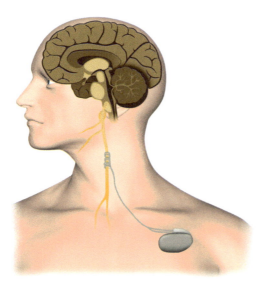

Figure 8.3.2 Implanted vagus nerve stimulation device. VNS nerve stimulation by Alila medical media. https://stock.adobe.com/contributor/200850923/alila-medical-media

There are several modes on the VNS:

- **Normal mode:** Regular pulses of electrical energy are sent to the brain in cycles (segments of time when the pulses are "on" or "off") with the goal of preventing seizures. This is the mode the device operates most of the time.
- **Magnet mode:** A specific magnet (typically kept on the individual's or caregiver's wrist for easy access) is swiped over the device during a seizure to provide additional pulses of electrical energy to stop an active seizure.
- **AutoStim (or autostimulation) mode:** This mode provides additional pulses when the individual's heart rate rapidly goes above certain parameters. Evidence shows that about 82 percent of individuals experience an increase in heart rate with a seizure.[239] Unlike exercise and other activities that cause a more gradual increase in heart rate, seizures cause a rapid increase, which the device detects. Therefore, not all instances of increased heart rate will activate the device. It is possible that the device may generate pulses during other instances

of increased heart rate, which are not seizures. If the individual suspects this is occurring, the parameters may be adjusted by the medical professional.

The parameters for each mode are personalized after the device is implanted. Medical professionals can then program the device to set and change the parameters for the individual, or turn the device off and on, when needed. It stores information such as heart rate, number and frequency of pulses sent, and which mode it is in.

It might take one year of neuromodulation with VNS for the individual to experience improved seizure control. An individual with a VNS is considered a "responder" to the treatment when seizure frequency is reduced by at least 50 percent.[239]

The battery in the device may last five to six years after which it will need to be changed, requiring additional surgery.

Studies show that in individuals who undergo VNS treatment:

- 23 to 57 percent of children and adults with drug-resistant epilepsy achieve responder status.[239]
- 8 percent of individuals achieve complete seizure freedom within 24 to 48 months.[239]
- Improvements in quality of life, such as alertness and mood are demonstrated.[240]
- Reduced rates of sudden unexpected death in epilepsy (SUDEP) are displayed.[239]

Adverse side effects from VNS treatment may occur, such as a tingling or mild discomfort in the neck or a prickly feeling on the skin.[241] Due to the proximity of the vocal cords to the vagus nerve, vocal cord paralysis, hoarseness, sore throat, or cough may occur, but usually this improves with time and by adjusting the VNS parameters.[239,242] Additional adverse side effects such as infection at the implantation site or the development of a hematoma (a large collection of blood under the skin resulting in swelling and discoloration) occur in about 9 percent of individuals after VNS surgery.[239] Some individuals may experience cardiac arrhythmias during or immediately after VNS surgery.[239]

Individuals with VNS should not have therapeutic ultrasounds (ultrasounds done during physical therapy or used to promote healing). These might create heat in the VNS system, which could damage the device. Diagnostic ultrasounds are fine as they do not generate heat, but MRI imaging of some body parts (i.e., those near the VNS device and electrodes) should not be done.[241] It is important to inform medical professionals of the device before any imaging is done. Metal detectors, such as those used at airports, may sound an alarm with VNS. Handheld detector devices are also not recommended, and airport security should be asked to not use these and instead perform a visual inspection or a pat-down search.[243]

b) Responsive neurostimulation

The responsive neurostimulation (RNS) device is surgically implanted to monitor for unusual electrical activity in the brain and send electrical stimulation to specific areas of the brain before a seizure begins or right after one starts. It is implanted under the scalp, in the skull, and electrodes are placed in specific areas of the brain and connected to the device with wires (also known as leads). See Figure 8.3.3.

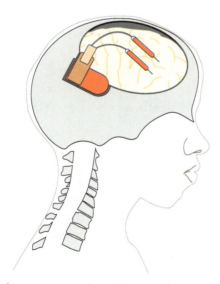

Figure 8.3.3 Implanted responsive neurostimulation device.

RNS devices are approved for use in individuals 18 years and older with drug-resistant focal epilepsy with onset zones in one or two regions of the brain in which surgical removal of those areas is not possible. However, research is ongoing to hopefully widen their use.[244]

The individual's seizure onset zone determines the placement of the electrodes, which sense and respond to abnormal electrical activity in the brain with a small pulse of stimulation. The pulse can stop the focal onset seizure from occurring, lessen its effect, or prevent it from becoming a focal to generalized seizure.[244]

Studies show:

- In a group of children (mean age of 14.9 years) with RNS devices, 65 percent were responders (those with a 50 percent or greater reduction in seizure frequency) and 10 percent were seizure-free at follow-up (mean time of 15.6 months).[245]
- In adults with drug-resistant focal epilepsy, the RNS device reduces the frequency of disabling seizures* at the start of treatment, and the reduced frequency is maintained over time.[246]
- Overall quality of life in adults with drug-resistant focal epilepsy is improved after RNS implantation without negative impact to mood or cognition.[246]

Adverse side effects from RNS surgery may occur and include infection, bleeding in the brain, product failure, misplaced wires (due to them moving out of place), and temporary weakness.[245] A study found that in adults with RNS devices, the infection rate is 4 percent, and subdural hemorrhage (abnormal collection of blood in the protective layer around the brain) occurs in 2 percent.[247,248]

MRI is possible with an implanted RNS, with some considerations. Parents or the individual with epilepsy should inform medical professionals of the device before any imaging is done. Metal detectors, such as those used at the airport, may sound an alarm with RNS. Handheld detector devices are also not recommended, and airport security should be asked to not use these and instead perform a visual inspection or a pat-down search.

---

* Disabling seizures in this study are defined as focal motor, focal impaired awareness, and/or focal to bilateral tonic-clonic.

c) Deep brain stimulation

The deep brain stimulation (DBS) device is surgically implanted to provide electrical stimulation into areas deep in the brain to prevent or stop seizures. It is implanted under the skin, in the upper chest area, and flexible wires (also known as leads) attach to the device and are connected to an electrode that is implanted deep in the brain (see Figure 8.3.4). This device is used in individuals with drug-resistant focal epilepsy.[249]

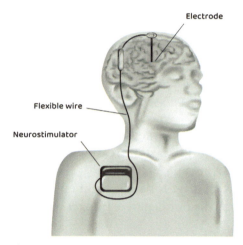

Figure 8.3.4 Implanted deep brain stimulation device.

DBS is generally effective at reducing seizures, though not all individuals with epilepsy will see improved seizure control. Implantation of DBS in children age 4 to 18 years reduced the frequency of drug-resistant seizures by at least 50 percent in 75 percent of individuals.[250] Overall, about half of all individuals with a DBS device will have fewer seizures, and improvement of seizures may increase over time.[249] It is not clear why some individuals respond while others do not, but it appears some types of epilepsy syndromes or types of epilepsy generally respond better to this treatment.[251]

Adverse side effects from DBS surgery may occur and include pain at the implant site, infection, paresthesia (abnormal tingling, burning, or numbing sensations of the skin), misplaced wires (due to moving out of place), and sensory disturbances.[252] Increased rates of depression and memory impairment have also been reported, although both are also known to be increased in individuals with drug-resistant epilepsy.[252]

MRI is possible with an implanted DBS, with some considerations. Parents or the individual with epilepsy should inform medical professionals of the device before any imaging is done. Metal detectors, such as those used at the airport, may sound an alarm with DBS or may cause the device to turn on or off. Airport security should be asked to not use a handheld detector device. Visual inspections or pat-down searches are preferred.

Epilepsy surgery

Epilepsy surgery is the broad term given to multiple types of surgeries, done with multiple approaches, depending on the type of epilepsy and seizure onset zone. In general, epilepsy surgery is the removal or disconnection of abnormal brain tissue or neuron networks to decrease the frequency of seizures or prevent seizures while preserving normal functions. Epilepsy surgery is performed in areas of the brain where seizures are thought to start or spread to. It may be considered in children or adults with drug-resistant epilepsy[253] and for other specific types of epilepsy, such as structural epilepsy.

Epilepsy surgery is a highly complicated procedure and is done only at select hospitals. The evaluation and preparation for epilepsy surgery is time-consuming, taking several months to perform all tests during multiple appointments and hospital stays. The goal of this presurgical evaluation is to ensure the individual is a good surgical candidate, identify the seizure onset zone, and plan for the specific surgery. Planning includes identifying the area to be removed or disconnected to provide the greatest success in seizure freedom, but also to have the least impact on normal function.[254] Sometimes, surgery is needed to place electrodes as part of the presurgical evaluation.

a) Presurgical imaging and testing

Imaging and other tests are often needed before (and after) surgery. Specific tests in the presurgical (before surgery) evaluation may include the following:

- **Invasive video EEG (VEEG)** involves surgically placing intracranial or in-depth electrodes (electrodes inside the skull, on the surface of the brain, or deep in the brain structures). **Stereoelectroencephalography (SEEG)** is a type of invasive VEEG that specifically involves the placement of electrodes deep in the brain structures and is used to more precisely pinpoint the seizure onset zone. Invasive VEEG involves placing electrodes while the individual is under anesthesia, and the electrodes remain on or in the brain for several days while VEEG is continuously recorded. Often, the individual will be in the intensive care unit or a specialized epilepsy monitoring unit during this test.

- **Magnetoelectroencephalography (MEG)** is used to identify seizure onset zones by detecting areas of epileptiform activity by measuring the magnetic field generated by the electrical activity of neurons.[255] This noninvasive test uses no radiation and involves the use of electrodes or a helmet to record the magnetic field.[256]
- **Magnetic source imaging (MSI)** combines MEG with other imaging techniques, typically MRI. This is used to better localize the seizure onset zone.
- **Single-photon emission computed tomography (SPECT)** measures regional cerebral bloodflow (rCBF)* during a seizure (ictal phase) and during a period of baseline (interictal phase) in an individual with epilepsy. A special substance, known as a tracer, is injected into the bloodstream, which is visible on a three-dimensional image of the brain, showing areas of intense bloodflow (indicating potential seizure onset zones).[257]
- **Positron emission tomography (PET)** shows the use of glucose (sugar) or oxygen in the brain. A small amount of a special substance, known as a tracer, is injected into the bloodstream. The uptake† of this tracer can show areas in the brain that are using higher or lower amounts of glucose or oxygen, which can help pinpoint seizure onset zones.[258,259]
- **Functional magnetic resonance imaging (fMRI)** can detect focal changes in bloodflow and oxygen levels that occur when an area of the brain is activated. It can be used to map cerebral cortex areas to help preserve motor, sensory, language, or memory functions and highlight areas in the brain that should be avoided during epilepsy surgery.[254] Undergoing fMRI is similar to undergoing typical MRI.

---

* Neuron activity is strongly correlated with regional cerebral bloodflow. Measuring this bloodflow can indicate enhanced neuron activity, as with a seizure.

† "Uptake" refers to how a substance is taken in or absorbed by the body.

- **Neuropsychological evaluation:** Neuropsychology is the study of the relationship of the brain and behaviors and how they impact each other. A neuropsychological evaluation, or testing, provides a comprehensive picture of an individual's current level of functioning to better understand their needs and strengths, and it should be done prior to epilepsy surgery to establish a baseline. This evaluation may also help pinpoint seizure onset zones. After surgery, the neuropsychological evaluation can measure the impact of the surgery on cognition, mood, memory, and behavior.[260]

b) Types of epilepsy surgery

Epilepsy surgeries that may be used in children are briefly described below. Not all types of epilepsy surgery are included. The field of epilepsy surgery is rapidly evolving.

The success of epilepsy surgery varies depending on the type of epilepsy being treated and individual response to the treatment. Specific questions about epilepsy surgery should be directed to the medical professional.

i) Temporal lobectomy

A temporal lobectomy is the removal of brain tissue from the temporal lobe on one side of the brain. This surgery may be recommended for the management of temporal lobe epilepsy, which involves focal onset seizures arising from the medial temporal lobe.[261] The medial temporal lobe is a specific part of the temporal lobe, which contains structures such as the hippocampus and amygdala. Focal onset seizures arising from the medial temporal lobe may be due to hippocampal sclerosis (see section 3.2).

An anterior temporal lobectomy (the anterior, or front, part of the temporal lobe is removed) is the most commonly performed epilepsy surgery.[262,263] Seizure freedom was reported in 65 to 80 percent of individuals following temporal lobectomy.[264–266]

ii) Extratemporal cortical resection

The term "extratemporal" is used when the impacted area of the brain is not in the temporal lobe, but instead in any other lobe, and even in multiple lobes. A range of techniques may be used, including a lesionectomy (removing a lesion), or a resection (removal) of a larger area of brain tissue in the lobes.[262]

Success rates vary, depending on the area of the brain involved, the technique used, and whether the seizure onset zone is in one lobe or multiple lobes.[267]

iii) Lesionectomy

A lesionectomy involves removing a lesion (structural abnormality such as a tumor) from a specific area of the brain.[263] The lesion may be caused by injury or by specific syndromes such as tuberous sclerosis complex.[262]

Seizure freedom has been reported in greater than 75 percent of individuals following lesionectomy.[268,269]

iv) Hemispherectomy

A hemispherectomy is the complete removal or a functional disconnection* of one hemisphere (half) of the brain.[270] This may be used for epilepsy that results from damage to one hemisphere of the brain, such as encephalomalacia (brain damage in one hemisphere with causes such as perinatal stroke), hemimegalencephaly (congenital malformation causing one hemisphere to become enlarged), cortical dysplasia (failure of the cerebral cortex to develop appropriately), Rasmussen encephalitis (Rasmussen syndrome), and Sturge-Weber syndrome.[271,272] Seizure freedom has been reported in 85 percent of children with epilepsy one year following hemispherectomy.[273]

v) Corpus callosotomy

A corpus callosotomy involves surgically dividing the fibers of the corpus callosum (which connects the two hemispheres of the brain), effectively stopping communication between the two hemispheres. Corpus callosotomy may be used with some epilepsy syndromes, such as Lennox-Gastaut, and in individuals who have severe generalized atonic-tonic ("drop") seizures.[263,274–276] Typically, a first procedure removes about two-thirds of the fibers (known as an anterior corpus

---

* A functional disconnection involves removing only part of the impacted hemisphere while also severing the connection between the two hemispheres of the brain.

callosotomy). If seizures persist, a second procedure that divides all the fibers is performed (known as a total corpus callosotomy).[276]

In general, a total corpus callosotomy is associated with greater seizure control than an anterior corpus callosotomy, and generalized atonic-tonic seizures appear to respond better to this procedure than do other types of generalized seizures.[276] In children with generalized atonic-tonic seizures, a total corpus callosotomy prevents these seizures in up to 91 percent.[277] As well, 88 percent of those undergoing a total corpus callosotomy experience a decrease in overall seizures.[276]

vi) Stereotactic radiosurgery

Stereotactic radiosurgery uses focused radiation beams to target and treat lesions in the brain that are causing seizures.[263] Stereotactic radiosurgery may be helpful when the lesion is in a part of the brain where other epilepsy surgery techniques may be difficult or risky.[278] This surgical technique may be used in treating gelastic seizures with hypothalamic hamartomas, which is an etiology-specific epilepsy syndrome with onset in the neonatal period and infancy. In a group of seven children and young adults with hypothalamic hamartomas, six experienced a significant reduction in seizures following stereotactic radiosurgery.[279]

The hospital stay following epilepsy surgery may be several days to weeks. Close follow-up is needed, along with ongoing appointments with other services, such as physical and occupational therapy and neuropsychology.

c) Risks and potential adverse outcomes

Risks of epilepsy surgery include:[253]

- Bleeding
- Infection
- Delayed healing
- Brain injury
- Death (rarely)

Because epilepsy surgery involves removing or altering brain tissues, adverse outcomes are possible. These outcomes will depend on the type of surgery and the area of the brain impacted. Some adverse outcomes may be temporary, and some may be permanent. Adverse side effects or outcomes include:[253,260,264]

- Changes in cognition or cognitive decline
- Changes in mood
- Memory impairment
- Problems understanding or using language
- Adverse behavioral conditions
- Vision changes
- Loss of typical function

Improvements in clinical care, including more clearly pinpointing seizure onset zones while preserving typical brain function, have decreased the occurrence of adverse outcomes from epilepsy surgery.

8.4

Other medications or supplements

I am not afraid of storms, for I am learning how to sail my ship.
Louisa May Alcott

In the management of epilepsy, other medications or supplements can be used with the same individual and along with pharmaceutical and non-pharmaceutical management.

Medications

For epilepsy with a specific cause or for particular epilepsy syndromes, medications either in addition to or instead of antiseizure medications may be considered. These include:

- **Immunotherapies:** These specific treatments that alter the immune system may be effective in epilepsy with an immune cause when used alongside antiseizure medications.[152] They may include immunoglobulin and plasma exchange treatments, among others.[131]
- **Steroids:** Medications with anti-inflammatory or immune-altering properties help regulate the body's reaction to infection, swelling,

immune conditions, and other conditions.[280] The body naturally produces steroids, and when they are given in higher doses than are typically found in the body, they are called high-dose steroids. High-dose steroids have adverse side effects such as weight gain and irritability, so they are often given for the shortest amount of time at the lowest dose that will be effective. West syndrome may be treated with steroids.[159]

- **Adrenocorticotropic hormone therapy (ACTH):** This medication increases the body's natural production of steroids and is usually given over several weeks, often along with antiseizure medications. It is used in the treatment of epileptic spasms, which often occur with specific epilepsy syndromes, such as West syndrome.[160]

Vitamins

Vitamins are nutrients that contribute to various body processes. Vitamins are found in food sources and are also available in the form of pills, powders, or other substances as dietary supplements, which can be purchased over the counter without a prescription. While they are not considered medications or pharmaceuticals, some vitamins may be recommended by medical professionals in the treatment of epilepsy.[281] Before starting any vitamins, consult a medical professional.

Atypical vitamin levels (too high or low) may contribute to seizures or epilepsy or a change in response to antiseizure medications. Deficiencies in vitamins may have a direct correlation with epilepsies with a metabolic cause.[131] In these individuals, or in individuals with an epilepsy syndrome known to be responsive to specific vitamins, vitamin therapy may be prescribed. Vitamins used in the management of epilepsy include:

- **Vitamin B6 (also known as pyridoxine):** A particular type of epilepsy syndrome, known as pyridoxine-responsive epilepsy syndrome, is treated with vitamin B6. Vitamin B6 deficiency is the *only vitamin deficiency to cause or worsen seizures*.[282] Vitamin B6 supplements might be helpful with increased irritability caused from a particular antiseizure medication, levetiracetam.[283]
- **Vitamin B7 (also known as biotin):** A particular type of encephalopathy, biotin-responsive encephalopathy, causes seizures and can be treated with vitamin B7.[284]

Vitamin supplements are also required for individuals on the ketogenic diet and may also be recommended for individuals on antiseizure medications that tend to lower vitamin levels.[281] Vitamin supplements may lead to fewer seizures or may lessen the side effects of antiseizure medications, but the overall evidence regarding vitamin supplements in the management of epilepsy is conflicting.[281,284]

The following are some findings about specific vitamins and epilepsy:

- **Vitamin C:** Deficiencies in vitamin C are reported in individuals with epilepsy who are taking antiseizure medications.[285]
- **Vitamin D:** Levels of vitamin D deficiency and insufficiency are found in children with epilepsy.[286] Studies in children with epilepsy show vitamin D deficiency rates of 23 percent and deficiency and insufficiency rates of 49 percent.[218,286] Conflicting evidence exists on the correction of vitamin D deficiency and improvement in seizure control.[281,286] However, vitamin D supplements are recommended to prevent musculoskeletal conditions and fractures.[218]
- **Vitamin E:** Vitamin E contains neuroprotective properties and may be helpful in managing neurodegenerative changes that can lead to epilepsy.[287]
- **Vitamin B9 (folic acid):** When taken in high doses, folic acid may induce seizures and negatively affect some antiseizure medications.[281]

Medical cannabis

Cannabis is a plant containing the chemicals tetrahydrocannabinol (THC) and cannabidiol (CBD). "Medical cannabis" refers to the use of cannabis products that are prescribed by medical professionals for medical purposes. The use of medical cannabis for epilepsy has gained popularity in recent years.

While THC is known for producing mind-altering effects and is used in recreational marijuana products, CBD does not produce such effects.[288] Laws generally regulate what percent of THC can be contained in these products, particularly in the US.[289] The regulations covering medical cannabis products make it difficult to obtain in some areas.[290]

Further research is needed to determine the safety and efficacy of medical cannabis products for epilepsy. However, research shows:

- Seizure reduction, improvements in mood, and improved language and motor skills are reported with the use of oral cannabis extracts in children.[288]
- In children with Dravet syndrome, the use of CBD results in a decrease in the frequency of some seizure types.[291]
- In individuals with Lennox-Gastaut syndrome (age 2 to 55), the use of CBD results in a decrease in the frequency of drop seizures.[292]
- In individuals with tuberous sclerosis complex (age 1 to 57), the use of CBD results in a decrease in the frequency of seizures.[293]

An antiseizure medication known as Epidiolex contains CBD and is FDA-approved for the management of epilepsy in specific situations.[288] Other forms of CBD available without a prescription should be avoided as they may increase seizures in children. General side effects of medical cannabis products include weight loss, nausea, diarrhea, vomiting, poor appetite, and sleepiness.[294] Serious side effects, including status epilepticus, have been reported.[294]

Management of epilepsy using medical cannabis is changing rapidly with changes in policy and legal regulations, and a medical professional should be consulted before trying any of these products for seizure management.

> Emma's seizures continued throughout childhood, many times lasting a long time. We often had to use two rescue medications just to get them to stop. We had many trips to the hospital when she was young. Whenever we would give more than one dose of the seizure rescue medication, they would want to monitor her since sometimes the medication can slow down breathing.
>
> We have a variety of rescue medication options for Emma, some easier than others. We found as she grew that using the rectal rescue medication became more difficult because we would have to first move her out of her wheelchair in order to give them. This wasn't a big deal when she was little, but once she was bigger it was a challenge. Also, needing to have a rectal medication at school or out in the community was not always

practical. Now we have rescue medications in the form of a nasal spray and liquid drops that are given buccally (or just right inside the cheek).

We reached a point when Emma was diagnosed as having drug-resistant epilepsy. It was not unusual for her to spend days after seizures in a "snowed-like" state from all the rescue medications that were needed. These would leave her feeling lethargic and exhausted, sometimes for up to a week at a time, and that was tough to watch. These periods significantly affected her quality of life, leaving her unable to participate in the day-to-day activities she normally enjoyed. We met with the medical team to talk about options for the antiseizure medications. These included the ketogenic diet, which I had heard as being a miracle for some people with epilepsy, but eventually determined this was not the correct approach for us to try. Another treatment option presented to us was the surgical placement of a vagus nerve stimulator, or VNS. After learning more, we decided to go ahead with this, thinking that even if it didn't completely stop her seizures (though we were hopeful), it would at least make them less debilitating and improve Emma's quality of life

The surgery to place the VNS went well. Right after, however, it seemed that her seizures were actually happening more often. They changed from being more generalized to being more focal, lasting from 30 seconds to two minutes, and happening every day, sometimes coming on due to a startle in the environment (loud noises especially). Around this time, she also started having bladder and bowel control issues.

I took my concerns to the neurologist who reminded me that VNS generally improves seizures over time and these should get better for Emma. I really tried to be optimistic. I know the neurologist had told me that as Emma grows, her seizures would change—maybe that was what was happening. But the change coinciding with the timing with the placement of the VNS felt like it couldn't just be coincidental, and I was feeling regret about the VNS. However, I soon realized that even if she was having more seizures, it was clear they were much shorter in length and they no longer required the rescue medication that left her feeling out of it for days. She would still get a little worn out from a seizure, but nothing like when she would spend an entire week trying to recover, meanwhile missing out on all the fun things she enjoyed. I finally came to my own conclusion that the VNS was a good decision after all.

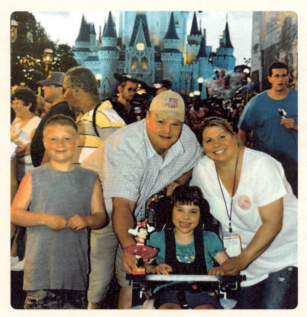

Family trip to Disney World: Jake, Scott, Emma, and Anna (left to right).

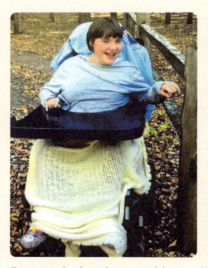

Emma enjoying time outside, age 18.

8.5 Alternative and complementary therapies

> Let us accept all the different paths
> as different rivers running
> toward the same ocean.
> Swami Satchidananda

Alternative therapies are therapies used instead of traditional treatment options, and complementary therapies are therapies used along with traditional treatments.[295] This section describes common alternative and complementary therapies along with available evidence presented, including cautionary statements when these types of therapies are *not* recommended.

Globally, it is estimated that between 13 and 44 percent of children with epilepsy use alternative and complementary therapies.[288] Their use is higher in low- and middle-income countries[296] where 80 percent of individuals use them, partly because of lack of access to antiseizure medications.[288] Alternative and complementary therapies may provide relief, particularly for symptoms related to comorbidities.

The reasons people may consider alternative and complementary therapies include:

- Hearing about a treatment option in the media (Internet, radio, TV, newspapers, magazines) or from well-meaning family and friends
- Wanting to try all treatment options in case the one they haven't tried is the one that works
- Wanting to complement or increase the effectiveness of the current treatment
- Wanting to relieve symptoms
- Believing the individual with epilepsy can do better

Often, alternative and complementary therapies are expensive, and any use of them should be discussed with the medical professional before investing in them. More importantly, it's essential to know if such therapies may cause an increase in seizures or may negatively interact with antiseizure medications. If the relationship with the medical professional is good, open discussions about these treatment ideas can occur. Parents, individuals with epilepsy, and professionals should be guided by the best research evidence available. This very principle guided the writing of this book.

Chapter 12 focuses on research and includes information on using evidence-based best practice in decision-making.

Minerals and herbal supplements

Minerals include substances such as calcium, magnesium, and sodium, which are present as ions in the body. Minerals and herbal supplements are considered dietary supplements. They are found naturally in food sources and may be purchased over the counter without a prescription.

Individuals who are taking antiseizure medications should have blood levels of minerals monitored routinely since some antiseizure medications may have an impact on them, and it has been found that low levels of some minerals may cause seizures.[282] Taking extra minerals is not typically needed, although sometimes a change in diet or mineral supplements may be recommended.[282]

Herbal supplements for the treatment of epilepsy have been in use for thousands of years, particularly in traditional Chinese medicine.[290] Compared to medications, herbal supplements are less standardized and dose variations are common, which makes it difficult to ensure consistency and evaluate effectiveness in groups of individuals. Many herbal supplements have been suggested as being effective in treating epilepsy, but data on this is lacking.[297]

Interactions between antiseizure medications and herbal supplements are a potential issue with any herbal supplement. Several known interactions may lead to an increase in seizures.[288] In addition, some herbal supplements may contain harmful levels of heavy metals, which may lead to toxicity, known to increase the risk of seizures.[288]

Diet modifications

The ketogenic diet is a recognized non-pharmaceutical management option for epilepsy and is described in section 8.3. A modified Atkins diet or a low glycemic index treatment are two other diets that restrict carbohydrates, but not as severely as a ketogenic diet, and both have been shown to have some positive effects in individuals with epilepsy.[298,299] However, aside from the ketogenic diet, no specific diet (e.g., vegan, vegetarian, meat-only, raw food, intermittent fasting) has proven to be effective in controlling seizures. Unless otherwise directed by a medical professional, it is best to follow a healthy, balanced diet. Any major diet changes or restrictions should be discussed in advance with the medical professional.

Hyperbaric oxygen therapy

Hyperbaric oxygen therapy involves the practice of inhaling 100 percent oxygen at pressure levels higher than typical atmosphere pressure, which is believed to help with neuronal regeneration.[300] However, studies have shown that hyperbaric oxygen can cause a decreased seizure threshold, meaning seizures are more likely to occur.[301,302] In addition, hyperbaric oxygen therapy occurs in a very small chamber, often only large enough for one individual and not conducive to providing rapid seizure first aid or assistance if needed. *For these reasons, hyperbaric* *oxygen therapy is **not** recommended as an alternative or complementary therapy for epilepsy.*

Other therapies

Other therapies include acupuncture, biofeedback, chiropractic care, yoga, music therapy, and more. As with all treatments, any alternative or complementary therapies should be discussed with a medical professional before beginning.

Key points Chapter 8

- The management of epilepsy can generally be divided into either *pharmaceutical*, involving the use of antiseizure medications, or *non-pharmaceutical*, involving the ketogenic diet, neuromodulation, or epilepsy surgery. Other medications or supplements including vitamins or medical cannabis may be used.
- One of the main goals of epilepsy management is to *prevent, reduce,* or *stop* seizures. Seizure freedom is the ultimate goal in epilepsy management, although this is not possible for every individual.
- Epilepsy in children often resolves, and about 60 percent of those with childhood-onset epilepsy achieve a five-year remission period and can stop antiseizure medications.
- Often, the first step in epilepsy management is starting one antiseizure medication, which is known as monotherapy. If different single medications are not effective, more than one antiseizure medication may be used together, which is known as polytherapy.
- Individual factors may impact the specific antiseizure medication that is considered and ultimately administered. These factors include the type of seizure, the type of epilepsy, epilepsy cause, epilepsy syndrome, sex, age, and comorbidities.
- Antiseizure medications may cause adverse side effects that often improve over time or may be managed by adjusting the medication dose. Antiseizure medications may also lead to long-term side effects and contribute to the development of comorbidities.
- The ketogenic diet is a form of dietary therapy that restricts the intake of carbohydrates, allows for a small amount of protein, and greatly increases the intake of fats to induce a metabolic state, known as ketosis, in the individual. The exact mechanism by which ketosis works to control seizures is not fully understood.
- Neuromodulation is the alteration (modulation) of neurons (neuro) and their communication networks with targeted electrical stimulation. When used in non-pharmaceutical management of epilepsy, it involves surgical implantation of medical devices including vagus nerve stimulation (VNS), responsive neurostimulation (RNS), and deep brain stimulation (DBS).
- Epilepsy surgery, in general, is the removal or disconnection of abnormal brain tissue or neuron networks to decrease the frequency

of seizures or prevent seizures while preserving normal functions. Epilepsy surgery is performed in areas of the brain where seizures are thought to start or spread to.
- Medications including immunotherapies, steroids, or ACTH may be used for epilepsy with a specific cause or for particular epilepsy syndromes.
- Deficiencies in vitamins may have a direct correlation with epilepsies with a metabolic cause. In these individuals or in individuals with an epilepsy syndrome known to be responsive to specific vitamins, vitamin therapy may be prescribed.
- The use of medical cannabis for epilepsy has gained popularity in recent years.
- Alternative and complementary therapies should be discussed with a medical professional before beginning them.

Chapter 9

Comorbidities of epilepsy

Section 9.1 Introduction 213

Section 9.2 Neurological and neurodevelopmental comorbidities 216

Section 9.3 Physical comorbidities 224

Section 9.4 Psychiatric comorbidities 229

Key points Chapter 9 232

9.1 Introduction

*You can't calm the storm ... so stop trying.
What you can do is calm yourself.
The storm will pass.*
Timber Hawkeye

Comorbidities are medical conditions that coexist with another condition, and there are many comorbidities that coexist with epilepsy. Approximately half of *all* people with epilepsy and approximately 70 percent of *children* with epilepsy have at least one comorbidity.[21] The ILAE framework for classifying epilepsy includes comorbidities as a consideration at every level of diagnosis (see Figure 9.1.1).

Comorbidities may be present before the epilepsy diagnosis, they may occur with the epilepsy diagnosis, or they may develop later.[303] Comorbidities may coexist with epilepsy by chance, or comorbidities may share the same risk factors or causes as epilepsy.[303,304] Long-term side effects of antiseizure medication or other treatments may cause comorbidities.

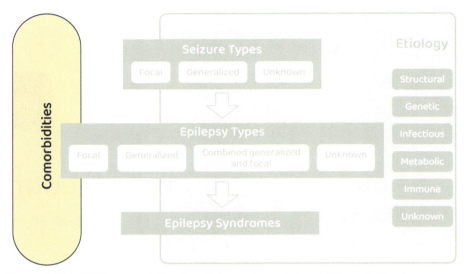

Figure 9.1.1 ILAE framework for classifying epilepsy. Adapted from *Epilepsia*, a journal of the ILAE. Used under a Creative Commons Attribution-Sharealike 4.0 International License. https://creativecommons.org/licenses/by-sa/4.0/

For many individuals with epilepsy, comorbidities may be more challenging than the seizures themselves.[32,82] Comorbidities may impact many areas and can be broadly classified as:

- **Neurological and neurodevelopmental comorbidities:** Conditions that affect the nervous system (neurological) and conditions that affect the development of the nervous system (neurodevelopmental)
- **Physical comorbidities:** Conditions that affect the physical functioning of the body
- **Psychiatric comorbidities:** Conditions that affect mood, thinking, and behavior

These are broad classifications and are not absolute; overlap exists. Table 9.1.1 lists comorbidities under each of these classifications.

Table 9.1.1 Comorbidities of epilepsy

NEUROLOGICAL AND NEURODEVELOPMENTAL		PHYSICAL	PSYCHIATRIC
	• Cerebral palsy (CP) • Developmental delay		• Depression and anxiety • Suicidality
• Intellectual disability, cognitive impairment, and learning disorders • ADHD (attention deficit hyperactivity disorder) • Migraine headaches • Sleep disorders • Autism spectrum disorders • Rett syndrome • Down syndrome • Tuberous sclerosis complex		• Musculoskeletal system disorders • Cardiovascular system disorders • Paroxysmal movement disorders • Autonomic nervous system disorders • Obesity	• Oppositional defiant disorder (ODD) • Obsessive-compulsive disorder (OCD) • Conduct disorder (CD) • Bipolar disorder • Psychosis • Tic disorders

Individuals with epilepsy and comorbidities will need the care of other medical professionals in addition to their epilepsy specialist. The management of epilepsy needs to be coordinated with the management of the comorbidity to ensure that one does not negatively impact the other.[303] Regardless of the specific comorbidity, the same principle applies: managing epilepsy with the comorbidity in mind, and vice versa, is of utmost importance. Coordination of care is essential.

Individuals with epilepsy should be evaluated for comorbidities regularly. This chapter provides a brief summary of the most common epilepsy comorbidities.

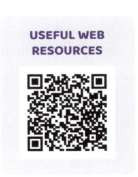

USEFUL WEB RESOURCES

9.2

Neurological and neurodevelopmental comorbidities

> Courage does not always roar. Sometimes courage is the quiet voice at the end of the day saying, "I will try again tomorrow."
> — Mary Anne Radmacher

Conditions that affect the nervous system are termed "neurological." Epilepsy itself is a neurological condition, and other neurological conditions frequently coexist with epilepsy as comorbidities. Since the nervous system affects all areas of the body, the impact of neurological comorbidities is often broad.

Neurodevelopmental conditions begin in the developmental periods (infancy, childhood, and adolescence) and interfere with how the brain functions, leading to issues including those that impact cognition, social skills, and emotions.[305]

Early interventions are shown to produce the best outcomes, and the management of epilepsy may help with the management of the comorbidities. Supportive interventions and services can help a child progress, which is why early recognition and management of neurological and neurodevelopmental comorbidities is so important.

While neurological and neurodevelopmental comorbidities are included in this section, some could be classified as physical comorbidities since they may result in physical problems, such as difficulties with motor coordination, delays in motor development, and challenges with speech.

Cerebral palsy

Cerebral palsy (CP) is the most common cause of childhood-acquired physical disability and is a neurodevelopmental disorder defined as follows:

> *Cerebral palsy (CP) describes a group of permanent disorders of the development of movement and posture, causing activity limitation, that are attributed to non-progressive disturbances that occurred in the developing fetal or infant brain. The motor disorders of cerebral palsy are often accompanied by disturbances of sensation, perception, cognition, communication, and behavior, by epilepsy, and by secondary musculoskeletal problems.*[306]

Data from the Australian CP register for 1995 to 2016 showed that 30 percent of children with CP at age five also had epilepsy.[307] A 2016 primer reported that epilepsy occurs in approximately 40 percent of individuals with CP.[308] Risk factors associated with an increased rate of epilepsy in children with CP include maternal hypertension (high blood pressure in the mother during pregnancy), cesarean section delivery, neonatal seizures, and severity of the CP.[309,310]

A majority of individuals with CP and epilepsy (70 percent) experience the onset of seizures within the first year of life, which is a younger age compared to a group of individuals with epilepsy without CP.[309] In addition, 43 percent of children with epilepsy and CP have drug-resistant epilepsy.[310]

Management: The management of the individual with CP is by a multidisciplinary team.

Developmental delay

When epilepsy begins in infancy and childhood, it occurs during an important time in the development of the brain, which grows rapidly from birth to about age five.

Developmental delay may present in any area but is most often found in:

- Gross motor development
- Fine motor development
- Speech and language development
- Development of social skills

In addition to developmental delay, in which certain skills are not developed, children with epilepsy may also lose skills that have already been achieved; this is known as regression.[211] The regression in children with epilepsy may be related to the frequency of seizures, the type of seizures, or the epilepsy syndrome itself.

Often, a major concern of parents of children with epilepsy is whether their child will meet milestones and if the seizures will impact their child's intelligence. It is important to note that a child with developmental delay can often catch up on missed milestones, and a diagnosis of a developmental delay in childhood does not necessarily predict adulthood capabilities.

Management: The management of an individual with developmental delay depends on the specific area affected and should be provided by the appropriate specialist.

Intellectual disability, cognitive impairment, and learning disorders

The following is an explanation of terms:

- **Intellectual disability:** Problems with general mental abilities that affect areas of intellectual functioning (such as learning, problem-solving, judgment) and adaptive functioning (activities of daily life such as communication and independent living).[311]

- **Cognitive impairment:** Difficulty with the mental process of acquiring and understanding knowledge.[312]
- **Learning disorders (also called learning disabilities):** Challenges in information processing, which result in academic difficulties or difficulties in how information is acquired and transferred to performing a skill.[313]

Thirty to 40 percent of children with epilepsy have intellectual disability.[21] Studies have found that:

- The age of onset of epilepsy, seizure type and frequency, cause of epilepsy, epilepsy syndrome, antiseizure medication, and genetic factors may impact intellectual disability.[82,213]
- Individuals with epilepsy with more severe intellectual disabilities have less success in becoming seizure-free than those with mild intellectual disabilities.[314] This makes achieving seizure freedom in individuals with intellectual disabilities particularly challenging.
- More severe problems with cognition may develop when recurrent seizures are present at a young age.[82]

Management: An important first step is completing standardized assessments to identify strengths and deficits. This may be done through neuropsychological evaluation, which provides a comprehensive assessment of an individual's current level of brain functioning in areas such as cognition, memory, visual and spatial skills, language and speech, math skills, and problem-solving.[315] Neuropsychological evaluation helps measure the consequences and impact of the comorbidities on brain function and how these relate to behaviors impacting many areas of life, such as occupational and academic achievements, relationships, and overall quality of life.[213] The results can help to identify appropriate interventions (including physical, occupational, speech and language therapy) and secure additional resources when needed (including special education services).

ADHD

ADHD (attention deficit hyperactivity disorder) is a condition characterized by an ongoing pattern of inattention, hyperactivity, or impulsivity impacting everyday functioning.[316] The symptoms of ADHD affect various neurological and neurodevelopmental areas, including cognition, behavior, and emotion.[317] ADHD may also be classified as a behavioral or neurobehavioral disorder.

The ILAE reports that ADHD occurs in about 30 percent of children with epilepsy.[318] Other studies have estimated the incidence to be even higher. ADHD is likely underrecognized, and a diagnosis of ADHD is often delayed in individuals with epilepsy.[82,318] Whether epilepsy causes ADHD or ADHD causes epilepsy is not fully known, but they appear to be risk factors for each other.[319,320] Signs of ADHD are often present at or around the time of the first seizure, and differentiating the symptoms caused by epilepsy from those caused by ADHD is challenging.[82,320]

Management: Management includes behavioral therapy and medication, often with medications known as central nervous system (CNS) stimulants. Conflicting evidence exists on the use of CNS stimulants to treat ADHD in individuals with epilepsy. Cautionary statements about an increase in seizures associated with CNS stimulants have likely led to some delays in treatment and undertreatment of ADHD in children with epilepsy.[317,321,322] However, a study concluded ADHD medications do not increase the risk of seizures.[321] The use of pharmaceuticals, including CNS stimulants, to treat ADHD in individuals with epilepsy is supported by the ILAE Task Force of Psychiatric Comorbidities in Epilepsy.[318,323] Most CNS stimulants used for treating ADHD have a relatively short active period allowing for a brief trial to inform the likely success of the treatment and possible adverse side effects, including any impact on seizure control. Non-CNS stimulant medications can also be used to treat ADHD.

Other neurological and neurodevelopmental comorbidities

Other neurological and neurodevelopmental comorbidities include the following:

- **Migraines:** A type of headache with moderate to severe throbbing and pulsating pain that is sometimes accompanied by an aura. Migraines are a comorbidity in 19 percent of individuals with epilepsy.[21]

- **Sleep disorders:** Conditions that include problems falling asleep, staying asleep, or unusual behaviors, emotions, or perceptions before falling asleep, while asleep, or upon waking up. Adequate sleep is necessary for brain development, and the disruption of sleep and sleep deprivation have been shown to impair emotional and cognitive functioning, learning, and overall quality of life, and lead to mood disorders and behavioral issues.[82,324,325] Sleep disorders are more common in children with epilepsy compared to the typical population.[21]
- **Autism spectrum disorders:** Conditions beginning in early childhood and characterized by persistent deficits in social communication and interaction along with repetitive patterns of behaviors, interests, or activities impairing everyday functioning.[326] Compared to the typical population, individuals with epilepsy are more likely to have autism spectrum disorder, and vice versa. Epilepsy occurs at a rate of 7 percent in children with autism spectrum disorder and 19 percent in adults with autism spectrum disorder.[327]
- **Rett syndrome:** A condition occurring almost exclusively in females, which is characterized by normal developmental progress until about 6 to 18 months of age, when developmental delay with regression rapidly occurs.[328–330] Epilepsy occurs in 60 to 80 percent of individuals with Rett syndrome.[331]
- **Down syndrome:** A genetic condition characterized by the duplication of chromosome 21 (trisomy 21), resulting in mild to moderate intellectual disability, slowed growth, and specific facial features.[332] Between 8 and 26 percent of individuals with Down syndrome experience seizures at any age.[333]
- **Tuberous sclerosis complex:** A genetic condition characterized by the development of benign tumors throughout the body, typically in the brain, kidneys, heart, lungs, and skin.[334] All seizure types occur in individuals with tuberous sclerosis complex and typically begin within the first two years of life.[335]

Emma was diagnosed with spastic quadriplegic cerebral palsy, which is a severe form of cerebral palsy. Dealing with this diagnosis and epilepsy sometimes felt like too much to handle. As a parent, dealing with two diagnoses creates a lot of challenges, but as you get to know your child, you start to be able to navigate those waters a bit better. There is no doubt it is difficult and at times overwhelming. I think that it's really important to remember that it is okay to not know everything (you are not going to), and it's okay to not have all the answers to which condition is causing which issue. It's easy to criticize ourselves as parents because we think we should automatically know the reason and the solution, but we don't. We are learning along with everybody else, and no parent should feel bad or ashamed for not knowing. That's part of the journey. The hope is that you will figure these things out along the way. But I can say that for myself, I have had situations with Emma where we never did figure out an answer or a cause, and although it's extremely difficult and frustrating sometimes, I've had to make peace with the fact that despite how hard I may try or how much the doctors may try, we are not always going to have the answers! My advice is to just take a deep breath, give yourself grace, and remind yourself that you are human and the same goes for your medical team. The answers will not always be there, but the questions will. Keep asking and keep moving forward as best you can.

As Emma grew and Jake met all the milestones she didn't, the gravity of the situation became even more apparent and really started to sink in. When you hear your child has a medical condition, it is difficult and painful, but in my experience, it didn't hit all at once. It slowly seeped in with every passing day and every celebratory moment that my son would have that Emma did not. When Jake started sitting up, Emma didn't. When Jake rolled over and crawled, Emma didn't. When he learned to say "mama" and "dada," Emma was babbling incoherently. Some of Emma's challenges are due to her cerebral palsy, while some are due to her epilepsy. Both conditions seem to impact some of the same things, so it's hard to always know which is the problem—only that they are both challenges.

My sister had a daughter around the same time as our twins were born, and she called me the day my niece started walking. Of course, I was happy for her, but I hung up the phone and burst into tears. Everything was bittersweet—wanting to enjoy moments for Jake and my niece, but also mourning the lack of these with Emma. I was mourning the child I thought I was having.

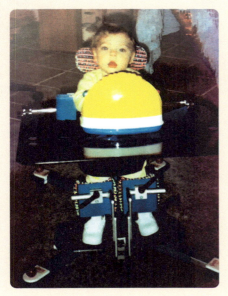

Emma using a stander, age 19 months.

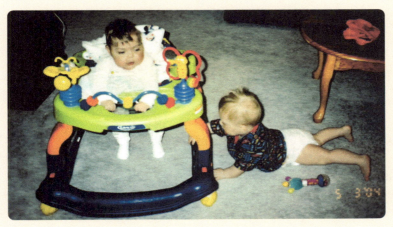

Emma and Jake, age one year.

9.3

Physical comorbidities

> Obstacles don't have to stop you. If you run into a wall, don't turn around and give up. Figure out how to climb it, go through it, or work around it.
>
> **Michael Jordan**

Physical comorbidities are conditions that affect the physical functioning of the body.

Musculoskeletal system disorders

The musculoskeletal system refers to both the muscles (musculo) and bones (skeletal) in the body, and includes muscles, bones, joints, and their related structures. Overall, musculoskeletal system disorders occur as comorbidities in children with epilepsy at a rate of 15 percent, compared to 4 percent in the typical population.[336] Abnormal bone health is present in 58 percent of people with epilepsy between the ages of 3 to 25 years.[21] The risk of fractures is estimated to be at least double in individuals with epilepsy compared to the typical population.[217,337]

Antiseizure medications are known to cause reduced bone mineral density and vitamin D levels, both of which can impact the strength of bones and contribute to osteoporosis and fractures.[218,338–340]

Management: Management of epilepsy in individuals with musculoskeletal disorders is typically done with antiseizure medications. However, it is important to be aware that these medications contribute to some musculoskeletal conditions. Since stopping antiseizure medications is generally not an option, monitoring for musculoskeletal conditions through screening tests is important. DXA scans (dual-energy X-ray absorptiometry) are done to screen for osteoporosis by measuring bone mineral density.[339] As well, monitoring vitamin D levels is important, and taking vitamin D supplements and calcium may be recommended to improve bone strength, especially in individuals with epilepsy who are on antiseizure medications long term.[218,341]

Cardiovascular system disorders

Cardiovascular system disorders may occur as comorbidities in individuals with epilepsy. These include heart disease, cardiac arrhythmias, and channelopathies.

- **Heart disease** describes various conditions that impact the heart and blood vessels. It is present in higher numbers in individuals with epilepsy than in the typical population.[63] Persistent and repetitive seizure activity may lead to chronic heart damage. The risk of developing a condition known as "epileptic heart" (heart and vessels supplying the heart are damaged) increases with the duration of epilepsy.[63] Individuals with epilepsy are at an almost fivefold increased risk of a heart attack compared to the typical population.[342] Takotsubo syndrome (TTS, sometimes referred to as broken-heart syndrome) is a condition in which the heart muscle temporarily weakens and is not able to pump blood as effectively as it should. TTS is often caused by a surge of stress hormones and results in chest pain, shortness of breath, and other symptoms like a heart attack, but without blockage in the arteries. Individuals with epilepsy are at an increased risk for TTS compared to the typical population.[342]
- **Cardiac arrhythmias** are atypical heart rhythms that may be too slow, too fast, or irregular.[220] In all individuals, a known

relationship exists between the electrical activity of the heart and that of the brain. A seizure's electrical activity may result in cardiac arrhythmias during or after a seizure. Ictal tachycardia (heart rate faster than normal during a seizure) occurs in up to 82 percent of individuals with epilepsy.[343] Ictal asystole is a rare arrhythmia, in which the heart rhythm pauses for more than three to four seconds during a seizure.[344] Individuals with temporal lobe epilepsy are at an increased risk of ictal asystole.[63]

- **Channelopathies** are conditions caused by an alteration in an ion channel.[345] Just as the brain has ion channels (which assist the movement of ions in and out of the neuron), the beating of the heart is also controlled by ion channels. Some channelopathies affect both the brain and the heart. For example, long QT syndrome (a disorder of the heart's electrical system) is a cardiac channelopathy (resulting from defects in ion channels in the heart) associated with some of the same gene mutations associated with epilepsy.[342] Long QT syndrome causes fast, erratic heart rhythms and may cause episodes of sudden fainting and, in severe cases, death.[346] Long QT syndrome may be mistaken for epilepsy and vice versa, or both may occur in the same individual.[347]

Management: Management of epilepsy in individuals with cardiovascular system disorders requires coordination with a cardiologist to select antiseizure medications that have the least effect on cardiac function.[52] For some cardiac comorbidities, a pacemaker or internal defibrillator is surgically implanted to control the electrical activity of the heart and prevent complications from arrhythmias.[63] Having both a pacemaker and an implanted neuromodulation device will require monitoring to ensure adverse interactions are identified and managed.

Other physical comorbidities

Other physical comorbidities include:

- **Paroxysmal movement disorders:** These are a group of disorders involving brief, involuntary movements and postures.[348] The movements are separate and distinct from any movement related to seizures, although historically, these disorders were often mistaken for seizures. In some cases, the same genes that lead to the movement disorder may lead to epilepsy, and abnormal brain electrical activity may also occur with both the movement disorder and epilepsy, making differentiation even more challenging. In addition, some movement disorder attacks may be immediately followed by seizures or seizures may precede movement disorder attacks.[349]

- **Autonomic nervous system disorders:** The autonomic nervous system regulates involuntary processes in the human body, including heart rate, digestion, and breathing. Comorbidities of the autonomic nervous system include gastrointestinal, respiratory, and skin disorders such as constipation, asthma, and psoriasis.[336,350,351]
- **Obesity:** Obesity is a chronic condition characterized by excessive fat deposits that may impact an individual's overall health. An individual may be deemed obese if their body mass index (BMI)* is above a specific threshold. Individuals with epilepsy have increased rates of obesity due to several factors. Seizures and antiseizure medications may alter brain pathways that affect hormone levels, increasing the risk of developing obesity due to overeating. Individuals with drug-resistant epilepsy, or those taking more than one antiseizure medication, are at even greater risk for obesity.[221] Activity restrictions, psychosocial issues, and lower rates of involvement in sports may also contribute to increased rates of obesity.[221]

> From the moment Emma was born, sleeping has been one of the most trying and challenging issues we have faced as a family. As you can imagine, or maybe already know, when your child has sleep issues, it tends to affect everyone in the family. Nothing in the household seems to function quite right without adequate sleep. We have spent many hard days and nights just desperate for sleep. Not only for us, but of course for Emma! When she would sleep too little, her seizures would get worse. Ironically, sleeping too much also caused seizures for Emma. We just couldn't seem to find the balance. After a particularly tough stretch of Emma (and us) not sleeping for more than about two hours in four days, I broke. I couldn't take it anymore and started sobbing uncontrollably. I felt helpless. Scott took me by both shoulders and said. "That's it. We can't do this anymore. We're taking her to the hospital. There's nowhere to turn."

---

* BMI is calculated by dividing an individual's body mass in kilograms by the square of their body height in meters.

That night Emma finally got the help she (and we) needed. She saw a sleep specialist and had a sleep study confirming what we already knew—she was not sleeping enough. After that, we were referred to a psychiatrist to help manage Emma's sleep with medications. And they worked! We finally slept. I still tell Emma's psychiatrist that she is an angel in disguise. Granted, we still don't get a full eight hours of uninterrupted sleep, but the chunks of time we do get are such a relief. We are finally to the point where, unless Emma is ill or having some other physical issues (cramping muscles and so forth), she sleeps most of the time fairly well. I still get up in the night to turn her over and reposition her so she isn't sleeping in the same spot all night, but life sure has improved from how it was. I think she would agree!

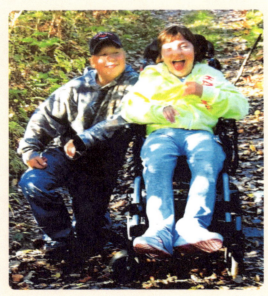

Jake and Emma, age 14.

9.4

Psychiatric comorbidities

Out of your vulnerabilities will come your strength.
Sigmund Freud

Psychiatric comorbidities affect mood, thinking, and behavior. They may also be called mental health or behavioral disorders. They are one of the most common comorbid conditions in epilepsy, with psychiatric and behavioral problems reported in 35 to 50 percent of children with epilepsy.[318] This is seven- to tenfold higher than in the general population.[21]

Depression and anxiety

Depression is a disorder characterized by a persistent decreased mood, lack of interest in activities, or loss of pleasure.[352] Anxiety is a disorder characterized by persistent feelings of worry and tension.[353] Depression and anxiety often occur together and are common in individuals with epilepsy. In children and adolescents with epilepsy, depression occurs in 14 percent and anxiety in 19 percent.[354] By contrast, the Centers for Disease Control (CDC) notes that in the US, in children and adolescents (age 3 to 17) the rate of depression is 4 percent, and the rate of anxiety is 10 percent.[355]

Depending on the cause of epilepsy and the location of seizures in the brain, damage to emotional centers that control mood can contribute to depression and anxiety.[356] In children and adolescents with epilepsy, contributing factors such as persistent seizures, cognitive impairment, language impairment, and intellectual disability appear to impact the occurrence of depression and anxiety, with those with more severe impact to these areas having increased rates of both depression and anxiety.[357] Lastly, concern about having a seizure in public, fear about talking about seizures with others, talking about the diagnosis of epilepsy, or fear of being away from a caregiver at the time of a seizure may contribute to depression and anxiety in children and adolescents with epilepsy.[182]

Suicidality

The term "suicidality" encompasses thoughts of suicide (suicidal ideation), self-harm or suicidal behavior, or completed suicide.[358] Antiseizure medications may increase thoughts of suicide, though this varies depending on the medication, and some newer antiseizure medications appear to have lower associated suicide risks.[216,359] Suicidal ideation occurs in children and adolescents with epilepsy at a rate of 14 to 27 percent.[182] Individuals with epilepsy have higher rates of suicidality and suicide attempts than those in the general population, and rates of death by suicide are higher in individuals with epilepsy.[216,358]

Other psychiatric comorbidities include the following:

- **Oppositional defiant disorder (ODD):** Characterized by the inability to control self, including emotions and behaviors. Individuals with ODD often have persistent angry moods and are argumentative or defiant.[360] Children and adolescents with epilepsy experience ODD at a rate of 13 percent compared to 2 percent in the typical population.[215]
- **Obsessive-compulsive disorder (OCD):** Characterized by intrusive or unwanted thoughts and a compulsion to perform repetitive actions.[361] Individuals with epilepsy appear to be at an increased

risk for developing OCD, particularly those individuals with seizures in the temporal or frontal lobe.[362]
- **Conduct disorder (CD):** Characterized by a persistent pattern of aggression, destruction of property, and rule violation.[363] CD occurs at a higher rate in individuals with epilepsy (16 percent) compared to the typical population (3 percent).[364]
- **Bipolar disorder and psychosis:** Characterized by extreme mood swings (bipolar disorder) or loss of contact with reality (psychosis). Bipolar disorder and psychosis appear to occur at higher rates in individuals with epilepsy compared to the typical population.[182,365]
- **Tic disorders:** Characterized by sudden, repetitive movements or sounds. Tic disorders appear to occur at higher rates in individuals with epilepsy compared to the typical population.[366]

Management: Recognition and diagnosis is an important first step in the management of psychiatric disorders. Depression and anxiety are often undetected and undertreated in individuals with epilepsy. Increased assessments at frequent intervals and with standardized screening tools is recommended.[182,337] Seizure control impacts the prevalence of psychiatric disorders. Depression and anxiety are more common in children with persistent seizures compared to those with well-controlled epilepsy.[357] However, some antiseizure medications have depression and anxiety as adverse side effects.[357] Antiseizure medications can exacerbate depression and anxiety or other psychiatric disorders.[215,216] Close monitoring of adverse side effects is important with a goal of optimal seizure control without creating or increasing psychiatric symptoms.

Key points Chapter 9

- Comorbidities are other medical conditions that coexist with another condition. Many comorbidities coexist with epilepsy. Approximately half of all people with epilepsy have at least one comorbidity, and approximately 70 percent of children with epilepsy have at least one comorbidity.
- Comorbidities may be present before the epilepsy diagnosis, occur with the epilepsy diagnosis, or develop later. Comorbidities may coexist with epilepsy by chance, or comorbidities and epilepsy may share the same risk factors or causes as epilepsy.
- Comorbidities may impact many areas and can be broadly classified as neurological and neurodevelopmental, physical, and psychiatric.
- For many individuals with epilepsy, comorbidities may be more challenging than the seizures themselves.
- Additional specialist evaluations are often needed to diagnose, manage, and treat comorbidities. The management of epilepsy should be coordinated with the management of the comorbidity to ensure management of one does not negatively impact the other.

Chapter 10

Growing up with epilepsy

Section 10.1 Introduction 235
Section 10.2 Psychosocial impact of epilepsy 236
Section 10.3 Activity modifications and lifestyle considerations 238
Section 10.4 Education and career planning 245
Section 10.5 Transition to adult care 249
Section 10.6 Family planning and pregnancy 253
Key points Chapter 10 258

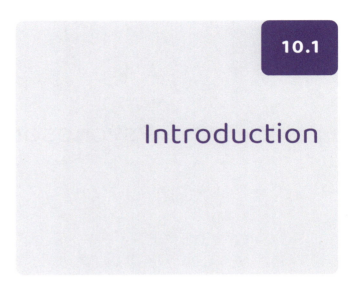

10.1 Introduction

He who conquers himself is the mightiest warrior.
Confucious

This chapter addresses growing up with an epilepsy diagnosis. It includes the psychosocial impact of epilepsy, acknowledging and understanding activity modifications and lifestyle considerations, education and career planning, transitioning from pediatric to adult care, and family planning and pregnancy considerations. While this chapter addresses topics in general, it's important to remember that every individual with epilepsy has a different experience.

Throughout life, working closely with relevant medical professionals is important as an individual with epilepsy may experience different challenges as they grow.

USEFUL WEB RESOURCES

10.2 Psychosocial impact of epilepsy

> I've learned that people will forget what you said, people will forget what you did, but people will never forget how you made them feel.
>
> Maya Angelou

The psychosocial impact of a condition refers to how the condition affects a person's emotions, mental health, relationships, and ability to interact with others in daily life. The psychosocial impact of epilepsy may include issues with peers, such as bullying and teasing, or individual challenges, such as loss of self-esteem and confidence.[367] Children may be afraid of having a seizure and may not feel comfortable talking with others about their seizures. Fear of being away from parents when a seizure happens may also lead to separation anxiety.[182] Restrictions may be placed on individuals with epilepsy, limiting their independence. Inability to do things that peers can do, such as driving, playing sports, or swimming, may negatively impact social relationships.[368] When seizures are controlled and children can more actively participate in activities such as sports, overall quality of life is increased.[369] Overrestriction of activities is associated with negative peer interactions and poor self-esteem.[32]

Helping individuals, especially children, know what to say to others about their epilepsy can help empower them not to be embarrassed or ashamed of their condition. Increasing education about epilepsy has been shown to decrease negative attitudes toward epilepsy,[370] and educating others about epilepsy, particularly classmates, may help decrease the stigma associated with this condition.[21]

It is also important to remember that comorbidities, addressed in the previous chapter, may also have a psychosocial impact on the individual.

10.3 Activity modifications and lifestyle considerations

Know your limits, but never stop trying to exceed them.
Unknown

A diagnosis of epilepsy can impact a person's activities and lifestyle, primarily due to risk of injury related to seizures. Population-based studies from multiple countries have found that both children and adults with epilepsy are at increased risk of accidental injury compared to the typical population.[191,371–373] This includes an 18 percent increased risk of fracture and a 49 percent increased risk of burns[371] and is affected by factors such as seizure frequency[372] and the presence of comorbidities.[191]

In addition, children and young adults with epilepsy are more than twice as likely to experience medicinal poisoning compared to the general population, particularly for those between 19 and 24 years of age. This risk includes intentional or unintentional overdosing and attempts at self-harm with medications (either antiseizure medications or other medications).[371]

It is important, therefore, for parents of children with epilepsy, and the individuals themselves, to be aware of activities that may put them at

10.3 ACTIVITY MODIFICATIONS AND LIFESTYLE CONSIDERATIONS

increased risk of accidental injury. Some individuals may be advised to modify or restrict certain activities to reduce this risk.

This section covers some, though not all, activities impacted by epilepsy. Safety tips are included where relevant, but specific strategies to decrease risk should be discussed with a medical professional. Areas included are:

- Driving
- Physical activities and sports
- Activities involving water, heights, and fire
- Using power tools and heavy equipment

Driving

In many cultures, learning to drive is a rite of passage for adolescents. Adolescents with epilepsy, however, may be disappointed to learn regulations for driving for those with epilepsy are strict. Medical professionals may be required to report individuals with epilepsy to licensing agencies. In the US, individuals with epilepsy may be permitted to drive as long as seizures are controlled. Each state has different requirements that an individual with epilepsy must meet to be licensed, and most states have a mandatory requirement of a seizure-free period (3 to 12 months) before driving. This clock resets any time a new seizure occurs.[374] Data on the number of individuals with epilepsy who drive in the US is difficult to obtain since many states rely on self-reporting of an epilepsy diagnosis. Seventy-three percent of individuals in Canada with epilepsy have a driver's license, compared to 94 percent of the typical population.[375] A study from India found that 15 percent of individuals with epilepsy who drive report an aura or seizure while driving, and 18 percent felt epilepsy or antiseizure medication negatively impacts their driving.[376] Another study found a slightly elevated risk of motor vehicle accidents in individuals with epilepsy, noting that the risk depends somewhat on adherence to antiseizure medications and the length of time the individual is seizure-free.[377] In those who are not adhering to prescribed antiseizure medications, a twofold increase in automobile crashes has been reported.[375]

It is important to talk with adolescents about the need to follow treatment recommendations, including taking antiseizure medications and reporting seizures that occur.[32] With good seizure control and adherence to antiseizure medications, it may be possible for an individual with epilepsy to obtain a driver's license.

Physical activities and sports

Participating in sports and other physical activities can be an important source of enjoyment. As well, physical activity is important in maintaining health and preventing issues such as obesity. For most individuals, exercise is unlikely to increase seizure frequency and, in fact, a decrease in seizures and an increase in seizure threshold have been associated with exercise.[378] Individuals with epilepsy should be encouraged to participate in sports and other activities as much as they are able.[379] No risk of increased seizures is associated with contact sports.[378]

Table 10.3.1 presents sports that have been categorized into three groups according to risk level. The sports listed are assigned to a group based on potential risk of injury or death for both persons with epilepsy (PWEs) and for bystanders, if a seizure should occur during the event.[378] The three categories are:

- Group 1 sports (no significant additional risk)
- Group 2 sports (moderate risks for PWEs but not to bystanders)
- Group 3 sports (high risk for PWEs and, for some sports, for bystanders)

The categorization takes into account the most common conditions that are likely to apply when individuals with epilepsy participate in these sports. Some sports fall into a "gray zone," and there are individual characteristics or circumstances for which a different group would be indicated based on the judgment of the medical professional.

Table 10.3.1 Participation in sports: Risk level of injury or death for persons with epilepsy (PWEs) and for bystanders

GROUP 1 (NO SIGNIFICANT ADDITIONAL RISK)	GROUP 2 (MODERATE RISK FOR PWES BUT NOT BYSTANDERS)	GROUP 3 (HIGH RISK FOR PWES AND, FOR SOME SPORTS, FOR BYSTANDERS)
• Athletics (except for sports listed under group 2) • Bowling • Most collective contact sports (judo, wrestling, etc.) • Collective sports on the ground (baseball, basketball, cricket, field hockey, football, rugby, volleyball, etc.) • Cross-country skiing • Curling • Dancing • Golf • Racquet sports (squash, table tennis, tennis, etc.)	• Alpine skiing • Archery • Athletics (pole vault) • Biathlon, triathlon, modern pentathlon • Canoeing • Collective contact sports involving potentially serious injury (e.g., boxing, karate, etc.) • Cycling • Fencing • Gymnastics • Horse riding (e.g., Olympic equestrian events, dressage, show jumping) • Ice hockey • Shooting • Skateboarding • Skating • Snowboarding • Swimming • Water skiing • Weightlifting	• Aviation • Climbing • Diving (platform, springboard) • Horse racing • Motor sports • Parachuting (and similar sports) • Rodeo • Scuba diving • Ski jumping • Solitary sailing • Surfing, wind-surfing

Adapted from Epilepsia, *a journal of the ILAE. Used under a Creative Commons Attribution-Sharealike 4.0 International License https://creativecommons.org/licenses/by-sa/4.0/*

Table 10.3.2 further classifies the three groups of sports based on whether they are permitted, depending on frequency and types of seizures.

Table 10.3.2. Permitted sports for persons with epilepsy (PWEs)

	ONE OR MORE SYMPTOMATIC SEIZURES	SINGLE UNPROVOKED SEIZURE	SEIZURE-FREE (12 MONTHS OR LONGER)	SLEEP-RELATED SEIZURES ONLY
Group 1	Permitted	Permitted	Permitted	Permitted
Group 2	Permitted at discretion of medical professional with restrictions	Permitted after 12 months seizure-free	Permitted	Permitted at discretion of medical professional with restrictions
Group 3	Permitted at discretion of medical professional with restrictions	Permitted after 12 months seizure-free	Permitted	Generally barred but may be considered with restrictions at discretion of medical professional for sports posing no risk to bystanders

SEIZURES WITHOUT IMPAIRED AWARENESS	SEIZURES WITH IMPAIRED AWARENESS	EPILEPSY RESOLVED >10 YEARS OFF ANTISEIZURE MEDICATION	MEDICATION WITHDRAWAL
Permitted	Permitted at discretion of medical professional; applies when seizures are precipitated by specific activities	Permitted	Permitted at discretion of medical professional; applies when seizures are precipitated by specific activities
Permitted at discretion of medical professional with restrictions	Permitted at discretion of medical professional with restrictions	Permitted	Permitted after appropriate periods following antiseizure medication cessation
Generally barred but may be considered with restrictions at discretion of medical professional for sports posing no risk to bystanders	Generally barred but may be considered with restrictions at discretion of medical professional for sports posing no risk to bystanders	Permitted	Permitted after appropriate periods following antiseizure medication cessation

Adapted from Epilepsia, *a journal of the ILAE. Used under a Creative Commons Attribution-Sharealike 4.0 International License https://creativecommons.org/licenses/by-sa/4.0/*

Activities involving water, heights, and fire

Activities involving water or heights may pose safety risks to individuals with epilepsy. While swimming, individuals with epilepsy should be supervised, and wearing a life jacket is recommended. Individuals with epilepsy should avoid taking baths unless they are supervised; showering is a safer option.

Activities involving heights, such as climbing on ladders, skydiving, or jumping onto other surfaces without a safety harness, should be avoided, especially when seizures are not controlled.[379,380]

Individuals with uncontrolled seizures need to be particularly careful around open flames, such as campfires or gas stoves, and should sit back from campfires and use electric stovetops or the back burners on gas stovetops if possible.[380]

Using power tools and heavy equipment

When individuals with epilepsy use power tools and heavy equipment, such as lawnmowers or snowblowers, additional safety considerations are needed. Safety guards and automatic stop switches can improve safety and should be used. Protective gear, as needed, should also be worn.[380]

10.4

Education and career planning

> We all have different gifts, so we all have different ways of saying to the world who we are.
> **Fred Rogers**

In many cultures, success is defined by education level and career (occupation). Quality-of-life scales include occupational roles, material well-being, and financial security, all of which can be positively correlated with a higher level of education.[381] Career planning for individuals with epilepsy should include discussions about which careers could be pursued and which may be more difficult or avoided.

Additional resources for individuals with epilepsy often include support at school. Difficulties in learning may occur due to the fatigue and recovery time often needed after seizures. When children reach school age, it is important to involve school professionals and teachers in discussions about restrictions the child may have due to epilepsy. Everyone involved should have a good understanding of the diagnosis and the plan for seizure management, safety, and learning accommodations or special education where needed.[367] For children and adolescents with epilepsy (and other disabilities), often a formal plan is drawn up detailing the support and accommodation they need. In the US, legal plans known as 504 plans or IEPs (individualized education programs) can be helpful for children with epilepsy who also have learning problems.[382]

The US National Academy of Medicine recommends neuropsychological assessments at the time of initial epilepsy diagnosis and ongoing throughout management.[82] Assessments may also be useful prior to entering college or university to help a student with epilepsy choose a major suited to their cognitive strengths.[322] Unfortunately, factors such as lack of resources, geographic location, or cost may limit access to neuropsychological evaluation.[82]

Studies have shown that 73 percent of individuals with a history of childhood-onset epilepsy complete high school, vocational training, college, or university, which is lower than typical population data.[383] Further, a large study in Europe noted that employment status was affected by epilepsy; the rate of full-time employment was slightly lower for individuals with epilepsy compared to the typical population (70 percent compared with 74 percent), while rates of part-time employment were slightly higher for individuals with epilepsy compared to the typical population (15 percent compared with 11 percent).[192]

It is worth noting that:

- US federal regulations prohibit anyone with a history of epilepsy from obtaining a pilot's license. If the epilepsy is resolved, an appeal may be made for an exception to this regulation. Other careers within the aviation industry may be pursued.[384]
- Careers that involve driving as a main responsibility are impacted by the ability of the individual to obtain a driver's license.
- A career that involves scuba diving may be difficult if seizures are not controlled, and in some countries, individuals with epilepsy are prohibited from diving.[385]

In the US, the Americans with Disabilities Act (ADA) prohibits discrimination based on disabilities.[386] Individuals with epilepsy should be encouraged to seek accommodations with employers as necessary and should have open discussions with medical professionals about their risk regarding a career choice.

The Epilepsy Foundation has further information on careers for individuals with epilepsy, and a link to the website is included in **Useful web resources**.

> Emma attended public school from kindergarten through 12th grade. Although she missed a lot of days due to her epilepsy and other medical conditions, she enjoyed school when she attended, especially music. Emma's classmates all loved to be with her; in elementary and middle school they would argue over who was going to get to push her wheelchair through the halls, and whose turn it was to sit by her at lunch. They all had a lot of questions too. That was evident when we were out one evening at a favorite local pizza place. I noticed a young boy sitting with his dad at a table adjacent to us. He was watching Emma and he suddenly raised his voice and with excitement said, "Dad, I know that girl! Her name is Emma, and she goes to my school. Can I say hi to her?" His dad tried to quiet him and stop him from pointing and shouting for fear he was causing a disturbance, but I didn't mind. I told him he could come over and say hi to Emma as long as it was okay with his dad. When he rushed over, I smiled at him and said, "That was really nice of you to come over to say hello. Emma really likes her friends from school." He nodded his head and looked up at me and with really big eyes and asked with curiosity, "Emma eats pizza?" I smiled and said, "She sure does!" I assured him that not only did Emma like pizza but that she probably liked a lot of the same things that he did. He seemed so surprised, as if it hadn't occurred to him that he was capable of having something in common with Emma.
>
> Unfortunately, not all the memories are as pleasant. One that I'd like to forget, at the same restaurant, was when Emma started having a seizure. I jumped to my feet and tried to shield the other customers' view of her and take care of her. I noticed that everything got so quiet, and people were staring. We were on full display, and though I tried to ignore all those eyes were on us, I could feel them looking at me! I desperately wanted to be able to put up a wall so people couldn't see her, not because I was ashamed but because someone I loved so much was experiencing such a vulnerable moment with the whole world watching.

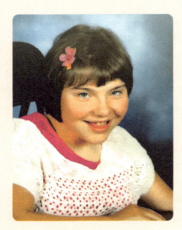
Emma, grade 4.

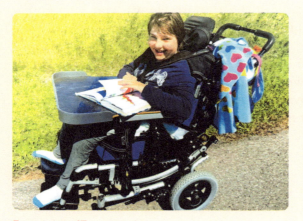
Emma, age 17.

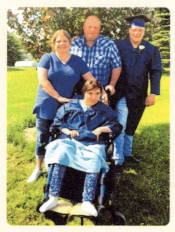
Emma and Jake's high school graduation.

10.5 Transition to adult care

*For in every adult there dwells the child that was,
and in every child there lies the adult that will be.*
John Connolly

Transitioning to adult care can be stressful, particularly for individuals with complex medical conditions such as epilepsy. The individual may have had the same medical professionals for many years. A level of trust has likely developed and the medical professional is familiar with all the complexities of the person's care. In addition, parents are part of the health care team: making important decisions, scheduling appointments, advocating and asking questions, managing insurance and financials. Moving into adulthood often means the young adult will need to take a more active role in managing their own health care.

This process of moving from a child/family-centered model of health care to an adult/patient-centered model of health care is often referred to as a health care transition.[387] A health care transition should include organized planning and education about the transition, assistance in finding an appropriate medical professional to transition to, and patient/family feedback on the transition. It involves more than simply changing providers (simply termed as "transfer"). Helping individuals to be as independent as possible is the overall goal in the management of children and adolescents with epilepsy, and therefore the transition must start early. Best practice recommendations are that this planning begin at age 12.[388]

Transition doesn't involve just health care, it also involves other areas such as education, finance, insurance, and guardianship. Figure 10.5.1 is a comprehensive look at the important transition questions: Where will I live? Who is my care team? How will I pay for things? What will I do?

Figure 10.5.2 Shows a typical form used for preparing an individual for transition to adult services.

When structured health care transitions occur, outcomes related to quality of life, satisfaction with care, and self-care skills all improve.[389] Got Transition is a US federally funded program focusing on improving the transition from pediatric to adult health care through the use of evidence-driven strategies for medical professionals, youth, young adults, and their families. The website has a lot of useful guidance, and a link to it is included in **Useful web resources**.

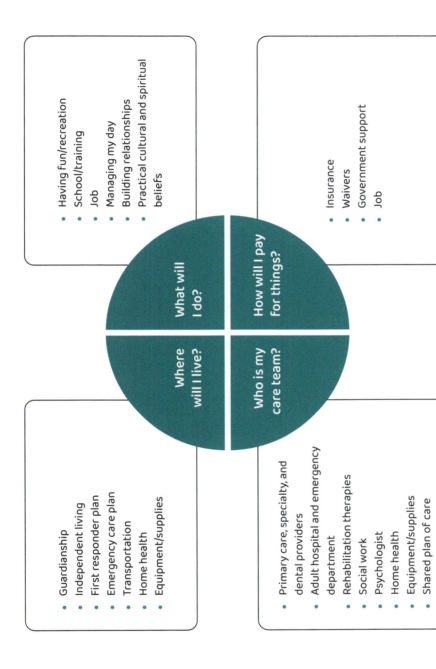

Figure 10.5.1 The important transition questions.

Transition Readiness Assessment Questionnaire (TRAQ)

Patient Name: _____ Date of Birth: ___/___/___ Today's Date ___/___/___ (MRN#_____)

Directions to Youth and Young Adults: Please check the box that best describes **your** skill level in the following areas that are important for transition to adult health care. There is no right or wrong answer and your answers will remain confidential and private.
Directions to Caregivers/Parents: If your youth or young adult is unable to complete the tasks below on their own, please check the box that best describes **your** skill level. **Check here** if you are a parent/caregiver completing this form. ☐

	No, I do not know how	No, but I want to learn	No, but I am learning to do this	Yes, I have started doing this	Yes, I always do this when I need to
Managing Medications					
1. Do you fill a prescription if you need to?					
2. Do you know what to do if you are having a bad reaction to your medications?					
3. Do you reorder medications before they run out?					
4. Do you explain any medications (name and dose) you are taking to healthcare providers?					
5. Do you speak with the pharmacist about drug interactions or other concerns related to your medications?					
Appointment Keeping					
6. Do you call the doctor's office to make an appointment?					
7. Do you follow-up on referrals for tests or check-ups or labs?					
8. Do you arrange for your ride to medical appointments?					
9. Do you call the doctor about unusual changes in your health (for example: allergic reactions)?					
Tracking Health Issues					
10. Do you fill out the medical history form, including a list of your allergies?					
11. Do you keep a calendar or list of medical and other appointments?					
12. Do you tell the doctor or nurse what you are feeling?					
13. Do you contact the doctor when you have a health concern?					
14. Do you make or help make medical decisions pertaining to your health?					
15. Do you attend your medical appointment or part of your appointment by yourself?					
Talking with Providers					
16. Do you ask questions of your nurse or doctor about your health or health care?					
17. Do you answer questions that are asked by the doctor, nurse, or clinic staff?					
18. Do you ask your doctor or nurse to explain things more clearly if you do not understand their instructions to you?					
19. Do you tell the doctor or nurse whether you followed their advice or recommendations?					
20. Do you explain your health history to your healthcare providers (including past surgeries, allergies, and medications)?					

Please circle how you feel about the following statements

	Not at all important	Not too important	Somewhat important	Important	Very Important
How important is it to you to manage your own health care?	1	2	3	4	5
How confident do you feel about your ability to manage your own health care?	1	2	3	4	5

© Wood, Reiss, & Livingood, McBee, Johnson, 2020

Figure 10.5.2 Transition Readiness Assessment Questionnaire. Reproduced with kind permission from Dr. David L. Wood.

10.6

Family planning and pregnancy

Your present circumstances don't determine where you can go; they merely determine where you start.

Nido Qubein

Family planning and pregnancy are important topics for individuals with epilepsy. It is important that discussions in this broad area begin in adolescence.[390]

Family planning

The World Health Organization states that family planning "allows people to attain the desired number of children, if any, and to determine the spacing of their pregnancies. It is achieved through use of contraceptive methods and the treatment of infertility."[391] Family planning for individuals with epilepsy is often impacted by their condition. Females may experience changes in seizure control based on hormonal fluctuations related to their menstrual cycle, and the effectiveness of hormonal birth control may be diminished by antiseizure medications, so other methods of contraception should be considered.[206,392,393] Further, hormonal birth control may make the antiseizure medication less effective.[393] Males with epilepsy taking antiseizure medications may experience lower sperm counts, sexual dysfunction, and altered hormone levels.[206,393,394]

As well, young adults with epilepsy who are thinking about starting a family may worry about what impact epilepsy will have on the ability to have a child or to take care of one. They may worry about the effect of taking antiseizure medications during pregnancy and the chance of children inheriting epilepsy.

A large study of approximately 500 individuals noted that females with epilepsy are more likely to express concerns about having a child with epilepsy when compared to males with epilepsy (73 percent versus 58 percent).[395] In addition, both females and males with epilepsy expressed uncertainty about having children due to their epilepsy (62 percent versus 48 percent).[395] Discussions with medical professionals about this topic are encouraged.

Pregnancy

Individuals with epilepsy are encouraged to have pregnancy planning discussions with their medical professional before becoming pregnant to help best coordinate epilepsy management while also minimizing any potential effects on the developing fetus. Seizures may increase, decrease, or stay the same during pregnancy, and antiseizure medications may need to be adjusted.[396]

It's also important to consider the already-mentioned decreased effectiveness of birth control for individuals with epilepsy.[390,392] The failure rate of oral contraceptives (one type of hormonal birth control) in women with epilepsy is 3 to 6 percent compared to 1 percent in the typical population.[397] Studies have shown that 79 percent of females with epilepsy report having at least one unplanned pregnancy,[398] and over half the pregnancies that occur in females with epilepsy are unintended.[390]

Some points to consider in pregnancy:

- Antiseizure medication drug levels may need to be monitored more frequently.

- Monotherapy, when possible, is preferred over polytherapy to help decrease the risk to the developing fetus.[396]
- Some antiseizure medications have a greater risk of causing birth defects than others. In most cases, antiseizure medications should not be discontinued during pregnancy as uncontrolled generalized onset seizures present a risk of fetal injury.[396,399] A link to the North American Antiepileptic Drug Pregnancy Registry, which provides information on the safety of antiseizure medications during pregnancy, is included in **Useful web resources**.
- Folic acid (synthetically produced variation of the vitamin folate, which is important in the formation of healthy cells) and supplements are recommended for all females with epilepsy intending to become pregnant. Low levels of folic acid have been associated with birth defects, and females with epilepsy have double the risk of having an infant with a birth defect compared with females in the typical population.[400]
- Infants born to females with epilepsy who are taking antiseizure medications are at an increased risk for birth defects, low birth weight, prematurity, low Apgar* scores, and respiratory issues, and may need to be admitted to a neonatal care unit.[401–403]
- Females with epilepsy have an increased risk of miscarriage when unplanned pregnancies occur compared with planned pregnancies.[404]

Despite a higher risk for infertility† and increased risks during pregnancy compared to the typical population, pregnancy and epilepsy can be successfully managed. Over 90 percent of pregnant females who have epilepsy deliver healthy babies.[396,405,406]

---

* The Apgar score is an evaluation used right after birth (at one minute and again at five minutes) to assess the newborn's health (heart rate, muscle tone, and other signs) using a scale of 0–10, with the higher score indicating more reassuring signs.

† Infertility is the failure to achieve a pregnancy after 12 months or more of regular unprotected sexual intercourse.

I recall about a year before Emma turned 18, a woman in the waiting room of Emma's clinic overheard me confirm her birthdate with a nurse. As I sat down to wait for her appointment, she approached me and said, "Oh your daughter is going to be 18 next year"? "Yeah, she is," I replied with a smile. "Oh," said the woman in a somewhat disappointed tone of voice, "that won't be much fun!"

She wasn't saying anything I hadn't already thought about. I recall feeling scared, nervous, and unsure of what types of changes would lie ahead.

Knowing what I know now, I laugh when I think about that day, and I wish someone had told me not to worry. So, if you are a parent of a child approaching 18, let me tell you—don't worry! It is not nearly as big a deal as it may sound. Yes, there will be some steps that may need to be taken, and depending on your situation, you may have to file for guardianship (that is what we had to do since Emma cannot be independent and take care of herself), but at the end of the day, there was really no shift at all in our eyes. It was the same family and the same Emma that had always been. Changing providers was a little different, which I compare to moving from elementary school to high school: a little less "child friendly" and a little more grown-up.

I want families to know that a diagnosis of epilepsy does not mean your life is over. It does not mean you cannot find happiness. We all face different challenges, there is no doubt about that. There might be days when all you can do is muster the energy to simply get out of bed. Just don't stay in that state permanently.

Raising a child with a health condition such as epilepsy may really make you question why things have happened. It's normal to want an answer. Sometimes we want to direct our anger toward something or someone. We might feel that if we can place this blame somewhere, we may feel less sad, less angry, less scared.

I have learned to stop asking why because there is no answer that will change my circumstances. I can't let the what-ifs destroy me and my family's life. Letting go of these feelings is a process, and I continue to work on this.

This life has incredible things to experience, and you have the ability to inspire others with the strength you show in difficult times. When you can find bright spots along the path and life, and you will, hold on tight to those moments and enjoy them.

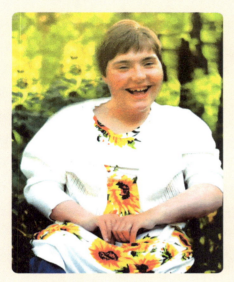

Emma, age 18.

Key points Chapter 10

- Throughout life, working closely with relevant medical professionals is important as an individual with epilepsy may experience different challenges as they grow.
- The psychosocial impact of epilepsy may include issues with peers, including bullying and teasing, or individual challenges such as loss of self-esteem and confidence.
- A diagnosis of epilepsy can impact activity and lifestyle, primarily due to risk of injury related to seizures.
- Individuals with epilepsy are often restricted from driving. In the US, most states have a mandatory requirement of a seizure-free period (3 to 12 months) before driving. With good seizure control and adherence to antiseizure medications, it may be possible for an individual with epilepsy to obtain a driver's license.
- Individuals with epilepsy should be encouraged to participate in sports and other activities as much as they are able.
- Activities involving water or heights may pose safety risks to individuals with epilepsy.
- Career planning for individuals with epilepsy should include discussions about which careers could be pursued and which may be more difficult or avoided.
- Additional resources for individuals with epilepsy often include support at school. Communicating with school professionals to ensure a good understanding of the diagnosis and plans to address seizure management and safety, and learning accommodations where needed, is important.
- A health care transition is the process of moving from a child/family-centered model of health care to an adult/patient-centered model of health care. When structured health care transitions occur, outcomes related to quality of life, satisfaction with care, and self-care skills all improve.
- Pregnancy planning discussions are recommended before pregnancy to help best coordinate epilepsy management while also minimizing any potential effects on the developing fetus.

- Females may experience changes in seizure control, based on hormonal fluctuations related to their menstrual cycle, and the effectiveness of hormonal birth control may be diminished by antiseizure medications.
- Males with epilepsy taking antiseizure medications may experience lower sperm counts, sexual dysfunction, and altered hormone levels.
- Seizures may increase, decrease, or stay the same during pregnancy, and antiseizure medications may need to be adjusted.
- Despite a higher risk for infertility and increased risks during pregnancy than the typical population, pregnancy and epilepsy can be successfully managed. Over 90 percent of pregnant females who have epilepsy deliver healthy babies.

Chapter 11

Living with epilepsy

> Nobody gets to live life backward.
> Look ahead—that's where your future lies.
>
> Ann Landers

In this chapter, people share stories of living with epilepsy.

George, age 24. from Minnesota, US

When I was eight years old, I was diagnosed with epilepsy. In the summer of 2008, I had my first seizure at a summer camp while waiting in the lunch line with my brother. I remember staring at the wall and then, in an instant, slowly waking up to see myself on a stretcher rolling into an ambulance. My brother was running alongside the stretcher, and I saw tears coming down his face. The first thought that went through my mind was that I got picked for a surprise emergency preparedness drill for our summer camp, and my brother was upset because he wasn't picked to be the fake patient in the stretcher. However, after the EMT told me that I had a seizure, I quickly realized it was not a drill.

The doctors explained to my family and me that it is common for seizures to occur during a child's development, but that children can outgrow them once their brains are fully developed. So I figured I was good to go. Unfortunately, one month later, while I was with my family on a beach vacation in Florida, I had not one but two seizures. (I also got stung by a jellyfish on that trip, which is not important but a fun anecdote to add to a not-so-great week for an eight-year-old.) After the trip, my parents took me to Gillette Children's where I was officially diagnosed with epilepsy.

I remember hearing that word "epilepsy" and thinking it was some kind of horrible disease, that my life would be changed forever and I would no longer be a "normal" kid. I was extremely scared. As a young child, you don't understand what epilepsy is. Instead, you hear the doctor say you "have" something, like it's a "bad thing." However, I learned very quickly that what I had was no "bad thing," and the neurologists and professionals were there to support me through my journey.

After my diagnosis, my nurse practitioner and doctor explained everything to ME. I think back on the first couple of meetings with my care team and how they allowed ME to make all the decisions, not my parents. I was thinking, "Not only do I get to dictate how I want to progress through this new journey, but I get to overrule my parents at eight years old? Sign me up!"

I was on antiseizure medication for the first two years after my diagnosis, and during that time I was fortunate enough to be seizure-free. My doctors believed there was a good chance I had outgrown my epilepsy, which is not uncommon for children with epilepsy. In fifth grade, I gradually transitioned off my medication. Unfortunately, five months later, while sitting in the audience of my school's talent show, I had another seizure. This episode demoralized me because it happened in front of all my friends, teachers, and classmates, and it proved that I had not outgrown my epilepsy. This was the first seizure that occurred in front of nonfamily members, so I was embarrassed because it was so public. However, through the support of not only my friends and family, but also my care team, I learned very quickly that everything was going to be okay.

Once again, my doctors asked me what I wanted to do, and I chose to go back on medication after that seizure. I am now 24 years old, and I am on that same antiseizure medication that I went on 14 years ago, and I have been seizure-free the entire time.

I still think about my amazing Gillette team members. They constantly showed me the love and care that any child needs during a dramatic change in their life. Throughout my epilepsy journey, they ensured that every decision was my own. When I started high school, my nurse practitioner asked me if I wanted to go off medication and see if I had outgrown my epilepsy. She shared her opinion and explained that there was a good chance I had outgrown it. However, I did not want to take that chance, so I decided to stay on medication. Despite my not following her medical recommendation, she completely agreed that it was my decision.

My team gave me the strength and courage to persevere through a difficult time in my childhood. They allowed me to choose my journey, and because of their guidance and support, it allowed me to "own" my epilepsy. It was no longer some weird disease that I "have." It is something I own and will continue to own for the rest of my life.

Today, epilepsy is still a part of my life but in the most minuscule way. I take my medication every day, but it has not limited my ability to partake in any activity I may choose. Epilepsy is a part of me, but it does not define me.

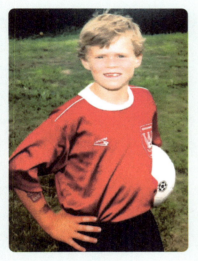

George, age eight.

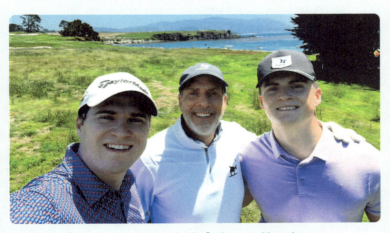

George (left), present day, with his father and brother.

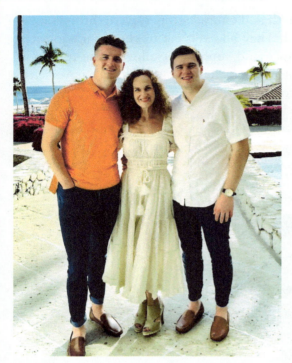

George (right), present day, with his brother and mother.

Sarah, mother of Nehemiah, age six, from Minnesota, US

Our family is only a couple of years into our journey with epilepsy, so I write with many fresh memories of what it is like to be on the ground through the early stages of an epilepsy diagnosis. When I was first asked to share my experience, I remember thinking that the only thing I can say is, "Get ready to pull all your hair out!" Thankfully, we are in the process of developing some more workable solutions than plucking hair strands, but it truly has been humbling to go on this journey and grope through the dark of many nights that held far fewer answers than we would have liked for our big questions. One thing that may make our story unique is that the hardest part about Nehemiah's epilepsy journey has not been the seizures. The hardest part, by far, has been the havoc that the epilepsy caused to Nehemiah's brain, and thus his ability to self-regulate and use language.

Nehemiah, my fourth child, was born in October 2017 through a natural birth process with no complications. He met all his developmental milestones with ease, to the point where we actually started him in his first year of preschool when he was still two (almost three). He had a fabulous time in preschool, and his teacher asked me toward the end of the year, "Is he always this calm and happy and well adjusted?" I thought about that question later, and realized, yes, Nehemiah is just so chill and always ready to go with the flow.

Later, in summer 2021, while we were in the midst of some preparations for a large event we were hosting, my husband and I said to each other, "Something seems just a little different with Nehemiah." It was very hard to put a finger on other than he just seemed a little bit more agitated and a little less focused. We figured it could be that we were extremely busy, and perhaps Nehemiah just needed some extra attention.

The busy season ended, and Nehemiah still seemed a little bit off. Later that summer, at the end of August, he experienced his first seizure. I was getting ready to walk out to our back porch when I heard some crashing noises coming from the bathroom. I ran in and found Nehemiah on the floor, very dazed. I had no idea what was wrong. I tried to stand him up and he kept slumping back down to the floor. My husband and I kept trying to talk with him and get him to look at us and stand on his own. Eventually, Nehemiah just completely stopped responding to us and his body went limp. It was as if he immediately drifted into a very deep sleep. We were quite scared, having never gone through anything like this before. We didn't have any clue about what was happening. We called 911 and the medical team arrived to give Nehemiah oxygen and do an initial evaluation. We were assured that his basic body functions were operating. The only responses we could get from Nehemiah were a couple of groans if he was poked. Otherwise, Nehemiah continued to act as if he was in a deep sleep.

Nehemiah was taken to a children's hospital by ambulance. Once at the hospital, he continued to appear as if in a deep sleep while many tests were performed. Finally, after about six hours, once they had put in the IV, he started to stir and finally regained consciousness. He had no memory of the ambulance ride. The last thing he remembered was being in the bathroom.

After the many tests all came back negative, the hospital staff said Nehemiah had most likely had a generalized tonic-clonic seizure, and his long deep sleep was an extended postictal phase. We stayed overnight at the hospital, and we talked with a neurologist the next morning. The neurologist explained that they often saw children around Nehemiah's age come in with a single seizure who never had another one. He said we could follow up with an EEG test at a later date if we wanted to, but that it wasn't necessary because he was hopeful Nehemiah would only ever have this one event. Given the neurologist's confidence, we decided not to do an EEG at that point.

In September 2021, Nehemiah started another year of preschool, and we continued to notice many changes in his behavior. It became harder and harder for him to sit still, and he had increasing difficulty with following directions, staying focused, and answering questions. As the school year advanced, our concerns became more pronounced. By the spring, we were feeling quite alarmed.

In May 2022, we were camping as a family in Wisconsin, and while our backs were turned, Nehemiah walked into a river behind our tent. Thankfully, where he entered was shallow and we were able to get him right out, but his lack of understanding of safety and his impulsivity seemed to have reached new levels of danger. I came home from that weekend and told several friends that something was really wrong with Nehemiah, but I didn't know what, nor did I know where to turn to for help since I did not know what was wrong.

Within a couple of weeks of this event, I noticed Nehemiah was having a lot of jerking motions in his arms and in his legs. In some ways it was so concerning, and in another way it was a relief because I thought it might be a clue as to what was wrong. I did some Internet research and made an appointment for him to see a neurologist.

Nehemiah had his first EEG in June 2022. We had only a couple of hours to monitor his brain waves, and I really wanted to know if the brain scan was "seeing" what I was seeing at home. Within that small window of time, the EEG captured at least 25 seizures. At that point, the neurologist explained that Nehemiah was experiencing myoclonic jerks and most likely had juvenile myoclonic epilepsy. I remember that I had a thousand questions, but the most pressing ones for me were not about managing his myoclonic jerks but about how to manage his behavior and keep him regulated and safe.

Soon after, we started Nehemiah on antiseizure medication. I was so hopeful that the medicine would bring back the Nehemiah that I knew, but unfortunately, starting the medicine coincided with a huge shift in his behavior for the worse. His agitation seemed to skyrocket along with his impulsivity. He would sit and just scream at almost every meal for no reason we could determine. I had to go backward in a lot of the care I was giving to him. We bought a stroller again so that he would not run away from me in the parks. Nehemiah had been potty-trained at night since he was two, but with the onset of seizures he reverted to bed-wetting. He could no longer sit still for a story. He regressed a lot with his sleeping patterns and woke up frequently. He seemed regulated only if he was jumping on the trampoline or swimming in the water. Other than that, he just seemed bothered and acted like I would if I had way too much caffeine and was simultaneously covered with poison ivy.

In addition to acting so personally agitated, his interactions with others and his language seemed to show more and more decline. He was treating the family dog and his siblings with increased aggression and continued to engage in unsafe behavior, such as running away. He was not able to respond to questions anymore. He often seemed aloof to life. Most of the time he seemed only able to communicate very basic needs.

We immediately started occupational and speech therapy, hoping that we might get relief from some of the daily difficulties that Nehemiah was experiencing, but the progress seemed agonizingly slow and barely noticeable. In July that year, Nehemiah had his first MRI with sedation, which showed white matter thinning in certain areas of his brain. It seemed unclear how this was also affecting whatever condition he was experiencing. This was the first of many visits to specialists, including a urologist, cardiologist, audiologist, psychologist, and geneticist, but none of them flagged anything too unusual. The full genome workup showed a mutation in a gene that is weakly linked to epilepsy and autism. However, it is a gene that is understudied and we were not able to draw many conclusions from any of these specialist studies.

In October 2022, we had our first overnight two-day VEEG study. The antiseizure medication had brought down the number of daytime seizures, but Nehemiah was still seizing quite frequently at night. In addition to having myoclonic jerks, he was also starting to have tonic seizures. Another antiseizure medication was added to try and decrease these.

At this point, everything seemed overwhelming. The language and behavioral concerns that I had had during the previous year for Nehemiah only seemed worse. I was also confused about his epilepsy. Juvenile myoclonic epilepsy typically affects kids in their adolescence from everything that I could read. And I wasn't finding a lot of resources that could explain the developmental and behavioral aggressions I was dealing with on a minute-to-minute basis at home. It almost seemed to me that I was dealing with something beyond just juvenile myoclonic epilepsy. We connected with the Epilepsy Foundation on a couple of occasions, and they were wonderfully supportive in answering as many questions as they could, but I quickly learned that epilepsy is an incredibly large umbrella and that the manifestations of the condition are vastly different. This made it hard to feel like we were even dealing with the same diagnosis as others whose concerns may be more about, say, frequent falling and impaired gross motor development.

We did a lot of research from the outset into epilepsy and started, perhaps as almost all parents do, seeking help through whatever means possible. We started B vitamins and fish oil and omega-3 fatty acids, not wanting to leave any possible avenue of healing unexplored.

In an effort to understand the dysregulated part of his behavior, Nehemiah had a full neuropsychology evaluation. Though he scored quite poorly on a lot of the assessments, they were hesitant to give him any official diagnosis other than "executive function disorder." Some of his behavior seemed like ADHD, some like autism, and some just the result of developmental difficulty. Because Nehemiah was still having some seizures, the neuropsychologist didn't want to label him with another disorder, given that his behavior could actually be the result of the chaos caused in his brain by his epilepsy.

We tried to start a third year with the same amazing preschool teacher, who only two years before had said that Nehemiah was the calmest child she knew. However, as he was no longer able to regulate himself in his social environment or focus long enough to not distract the other students, by November, his teachers were pretty clear that their school was no longer the right fit for him.

We were able to get Nehemiah tested through the early childhood screening in our school district. He was placed in a special education pre-K classroom that seemed to be well equipped to work with the kids who had similar developmental and behavioral challenges.

In December that year, we decided to start Nehemiah with a low dose of a medication used to treat ADHD. We were hopeful that it might improve his focus and dysregulation challenges. I remember being really surprised one night after he started this medication when he finally just played with his toys on the living room floor and imagined that the little characters were going to the hospital for an EEG. It was the first time I had ever heard him reflect on his experiences with epilepsy using language in play. His language had been so limited to only requests that to hear him process his medical journey through the voices of small Daniel Tiger characters (from a children's educational television show) almost made me cry.

If this medication had just had these encouraging peaks, it would have been a huge help to us, but the troughs seemed really hard for Nehemiah to regulate. His appetite was adversely affected, and it was very difficult to get him to eat. We stuck it out with the medication for a couple of months, but then decided it wasn't the right fit for him.

Another EEG finally confirmed Nehemiah was clear of seizures. He was still experiencing some EEG abnormalities (spike-and-wave discharge, slowing), but it was exciting to see that the medicine had indeed helped manage the seizure problem. Around that same time, Nehemiah's levels of his antiseizure medication in his blood were higher than recommended. The time leading up to that discovery, and subsequent lessening of the dosage, introduced another season of intense behavioral and regulation challenges. It seemed that he did not know how to hold his body in space without hurting others in his environment or the environment itself. I spent a lot of time grieving the loss of a boy that I had known, even as I was working to accept and love the Nehemiah who was facing this new reality.

At this point, when it seemed like any gains were impossible, I was worried that the antiseizure medication itself was negatively affecting Nehemiah's behavior, since when he started it, and when its dosage was too high, we saw a seemingly striking correlation to increased behavioral challenge. I wondered often about changing this medicine, but the fact that his last EEG had shown no seizure activity at all made it really difficult to feel like there was any option but to stay on it.

Part of what made life so tricky was that Nehemiah's dysregulated behavior seemed to come from nowhere. For example, one time we had gotten him to build some Duplo (large building blocks for children) quietly on the floor. He was enjoying himself and nothing obvious was irritating him. Out of the calm, he walked up to his brother, who was sitting quietly at the table, took his brother's art piece and ripped it in half. Out-of-the-blue impulses were happening constantly and I couldn't take my eyes off him. This made it very difficult to feel like I was giving my three older children the attention they needed and craved. I felt stretched very thin. Through all this time, I knew that Nehemiah had absolutely the sweetest heart and never intended to harm anyone; it just seemed as though his subconscious confusion was dominating his actions, and no parenting strategies I had used with my older kids seemed to work in response to his behavior.

Every night when the day was finally over, my husband and I would talk at length about Nehemiah and his care. It was becoming apparent that I would need help to care for him because he was getting more and more impulsive—unbuckling in the car, darting in parking lots, running to the neighbors without warning, screaming through every family meal. It felt very difficult to not have a behavioral diagnosis for Nehemiah because many community resources, including respite care of any kind, seemed reserved for children with official diagnoses. I reached a very thin place where I realized I could not continue in this way for much longer—we either needed respite help or a better diagnosis that could get us better answers or, preferably, Nehemiah needed to start improving. We began a season of intense prayer for Nehemiah's healing and simultaneous research into more help for him.

In March 2023, my husband and I started consulting via telehealth with a behavioral psychologist who worked out of New York City. Her specialty was kids with autism, which we did not think Nehemiah had, but autism seemed to hold the closest corollaries to his challenges with language, social interactions, and self-regulation. After hearing our story, she was very clear that there was no reason that Nehemiah couldn't regain the skills that he had lost. It was as if the behavioral regulation and language centers of Nehemiah's brain had experienced a level 5 hurricane from the seizures, making these centers formless and void. We began having hope that if we went back to ground zero and started over, we could make a lot of progress in rehabilitating these parts of his brain. We started following a lot of the psychologist's recommendations: we gave Nehemiah his own bedroom to escape the stimulations of life, we started practicing a lot of quiet sitting and enforcing stricter scheduling, and we began sleep training. My husband took the three older kids away for two weeks while Nehemiah and I exclusively practiced our new daily rhythms. I read some of the diary of Anne Sullivan who worked with Helen Keller's childhood behavioral dysregulations and language voids many decades ago, and I found that Anne's work with Helen was very similar to the work that I was setting out to do with Nehemiah.

Up until this point, I had been focusing on all the regressions that Nehemiah was experiencing as a five-year-old. However, I had to change my mindset and think of him as if he were 18 months old again. What would he need to know to succeed in the world at that age? How would I treat him if he was still a young toddler? How would I support his growth and language? These seemed to be helpful questions for me because they let me have a greater sense of agency. It was as if Nehemiah just needed me to re-parent him from a much younger age.

Also, at the same time as we were starting this behavioral program, Nehemiah was given the use of an AAC (augmentative and alternative communication) device through his speech therapist. I made a lot of very detailed auditory/visual schedules in his AAC device that were meant to reteach Nehemiah all the expectations for every transition in the day. I was very surprised by how he responded to this—it was as if all along he wanted to do the right thing but had lost all conception of what the next right thing was. The detailed visual reminders seemed hugely comforting to him, and he became very attached to following these schedules.

We began to notice some big shifts in Nehemiah's language and regulatory behaviors. It seemed like he was finally able to put into practice a lot of the skills he had been learning in occupational therapy. The AAC device also seemed to give him a lot more confidence with language, since he was able to use it to access all the words that would frequently elude him.

The language and regulatory centers in Nehemiah's brain were undoubtedly affected by the high frequency of daily seizures that Nehemiah experienced. But now, these centers in his brain seemed to have formed a positive feedback loop with each other, and the recent gains in expression and focus and language-based imaginative play have been striking.

Recently we were able to get an appointment for Nehemiah to see a neurologist at a Level 4 epilepsy center* for a second opinion. Learning more about Nehemiah's epilepsy has allowed us to make helpful connections with many other families whose stories matched ours almost identically. It was also reaffirming to hear that other families experienced behavioral declines in their child, especially when they were taking antiseizure medications. Meeting others going through a similar experience helped us not feel so alone.

We have a long way to go to get back to where we were before Nehemiah's seizures began, but we are now hopeful. We are still working on reducing the frequency of Nehemiah's running away and haven't made as many gains in this area as we would like. Some days all this progress seems so tentative, and I worry about the seizures starting up again and losing our foothold, but that will be tomorrow's challenge if that comes. I am trying not to borrow imagined troubles from the future.

---

* A Level 4 epilepsy center is the highest recognized level of epilepsy care by the National Association of Epilepsy Centers. Level 4 centers provide more complex forms of monitoring, evaluation, and treatment. They also offer a broad range of surgical procedures for epilepsy.

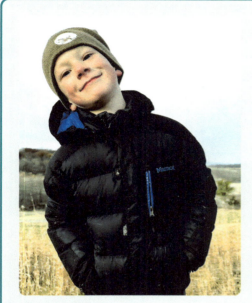
Nehemiah, age six.

Anie, mother of Missak, age 20, from Lebanon

Missak was about eight and a half years old when he had his first seizure. I remember it clearly—it was early morning, on a very cold day. When it first began, I thought maybe he was just cold and shivering. Then he became unconscious, and the fear set in as we rushed him to the hospital. I had heard of seizures and epilepsy before, but I had never actually witnessed anyone having a seizure—it was terrifying. At the hospital, he had an EEG, which showed seizures (epileptiform discharges, as they referred to them). He was referred to a neurologist, who talked to us about starting antiseizure medication if a second seizure occurred. Unfortunately, he had a second seizure shortly after the first, and he started on Depakote (an antiseizure medication).

While we were working to get his seizures controlled, I had a lot of anxiety and stress—sometimes just waiting for him to have a seizure. His seizures tended to occur about 20 minutes after he fell asleep, so naturally I would watch him sleep and even set up audio/video monitors so I could check on him throughout the night. I barely slept for about a year and a half, and my life became just that—monitoring my son. My work and everything else essentially stopped. Watching him have a seizure was the worst. I also worried about what other effects the seizures and even the medications may be having on him. However, I knew that I needed to stay strong as he had to have someone to rely on as he was scared as well. It was difficult for him to understand what was happening during this time—just imagine explaining to a child the concept of electricity in the head.

While he was on Depakote, he developed attention and memory issues, so he switched to Keppra (another antiseizure medication) and remained on that, despite continuing to have frequent seizures. Eventually, his epilepsy resolved, and we were given the miracle we prayed for. He is no longer taking any antiseizure medications and now just takes Concerta for ADHD.

When this first began, I felt like I needed someone to blame. For a while, I blamed God. Now looking back, I know that keeping my faith in this situation was the most important thing. I would tell parents of children with epilepsy to keep hope and faith, even in the most difficult times. Epilepsy does not always last forever, and often things can improve with treatment.

Missak has been seizure-free for nine years. I can sleep again, although the worry of motherhood never stops. Missak graduated from high school and is studying business management at university. He plans to manage his father's company and is working on that while continuing his studies at school.

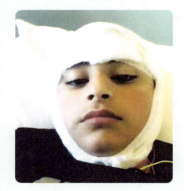

Missak during an EEG.

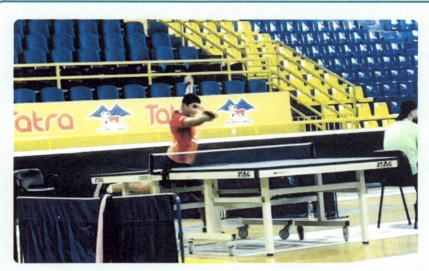
Missak playing table tennis.

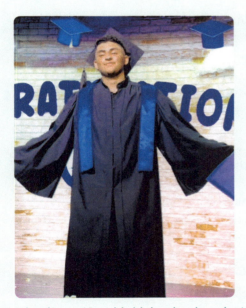
Missak, age 18, at his high school graduation.

Lisa, mother of Blake, age 19, from North Dakota, US

Lisa

Blake was diagnosed with DiGeorge syndrome[*407] shortly before his fourth birthday. That diagnosis and several surgeries were a lot to deal with over the next 12 years. Then, in the fall of 2020, when Blake was 16, something new began to happen. We started to notice little things, like him blinking his eyes a lot, scrunching one side of his mouth, or small jerking movements in his hands. When I would ask Blake about it, he would say, "I just feel kind of nervous." We weren't sure if this was all part of his DiGeorge syndrome or something else.

On February 1, 2021, we saw Blake's primary physician, and she referred us to a neurologist. I had just scheduled an appointment for a couple of weeks later when Blake had a major seizure. As a former registered nurse, I knew to turn him to his side and protect his head and body from injury, but nothing prepared me for seeing him stop breathing completely and turn blue all the way to his hands. We called 911 and prayed.

As we live 20 miles from town, it took 40 minutes for the ambulance to arrive, and by that time Blake was awake but confused. Instead of sending him in the ambulance, we opted to drive him to the hospital ourselves with a police escort. In the emergency room, they prescribed medication for him to take regularly until we could see the neurologist in three weeks. We didn't want to wait that long because we were concerned he would have another seizure, so we called the children's hospital we were familiar with (where Blake went for his DiGeorge management), and they were able to see him two days later. After meeting with the neurologist, Blake was immediately scheduled for a 48-hour VEEG.

The result was Blake being diagnosed with generalized juvenile myoclonic epilepsy, and with the help of the VEEG, the doctors were able to

---

* DiGeorge syndrome is a congenital genetic disorder caused by a specific genetic mutation. It can cause a variety of symptoms, including cardiac conditions, low levels of calcium, an underdeveloped thymus (a small organ in the chest that generates immune cells, protecting against infection), atypical facial structure, and developmental delays.

determine that the medication prescribed at the ER needed to change. With the new medication, his seizures were controlled.

The summer before his senior year of high school, after being seizure-free for six months, Blake was able to get his driver's license. He graduated in May 2023 and is now attending our local college for a degree in information technology. He also has a part-time job in the college IT (information technology) department. He drives every day but is sometimes still fearful that one day he may have a seizure. As his family, we sometimes are too, but we know that with proper medical care, medication, and by taking care of himself, he can minimize his risk for seizures.

Blake has a weekly pill organizer and marks his morning and evening medication on a calendar so he doesn't forget a dose. He wears a medical alert bracelet and always carries his seizure rescue medication. He also is not afraid to tell people he has epilepsy because he wants people to know how they can help him if he ever has a seizure.

Today, besides going to school, Blake loves spending time on computers, playing video games, and driving our side-by-side UTV (utility terrain vehicle). He's a pretty amazing young man, and I would know because I'm his mother!

Blake

I have epilepsy. I was diagnosed when I was 16. I must take medication every day, and I keep track of that on a calendar and with a pill organizer because sometimes I have trouble remembering. I can drive, but it still makes me nervous. I worry that one day I may have a seizure while driving. I never drive at night because the lights from passing cars bother me. I also have trouble concentrating and remembering in school, and I worry what would happen if I had a seizure at school. I have emergency medication and a medical alert bracelet that I wear every day.

I believe that God put me in the care of good doctors who really cared about me and wanted me to do well and accomplish my goals. I want other kids with epilepsy to know that they will get through this; just be patient with yourself and don't let fear get in the way of your dreams.

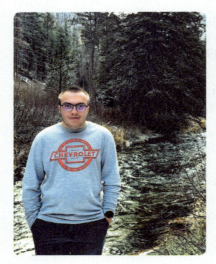

Blake, age 19.

Aline, mother of Charlotte, age seven, from Belgium

Our daughter, Charlotte, now seven years old, had her first seizure around age five, in January 2023. At the time, I was at home with my husband and our younger child, downstairs on the sofa. We heard groans coming from Charlotte's room. We immediately went upstairs and found Charlotte, who appeared to be asleep but was at the same time trying to spit. We tried to wake her up, but we couldn't get her to respond. She looked like a rag doll: her eyes were wide open, her pupils were dilated, but there was no response. After turning her onto her side, we called emergency services, all while continuing to try to get her to wake up. When emergency services arrived, they assessed her and found that her vital signs were good, but she would still not respond. She was taken to the hospital where she finally woke up and appeared to be just fine. The doctor felt comfortable sending her home, and I recall him telling me, "She's doing very well. It's nothing; just a little virus." It seemed that she had had an acute symptomatic seizure caused by a virus, and with that we brought her home.

A few months later, around 10 p.m. one day in June, Charlotte had another seizure that appeared identical to the first. She would not wake up, did not communicate, her eyes were wide open, but she was "not there." Another call to the emergency services and another visit to the hospital. Without being certain of it, the doctor told us the events looked like epileptic seizures. We still thought the seizures were perhaps caused by viruses as Charlotte had many viruses in a short period of time, and we hoped it was not epilepsy.

Charlotte spent the night at the hospital. The next morning, the neurologist came in and discussed epilepsy with us but said she would need to do further testing to say for sure. Charlotte was hooked up to EEG and taken for her test. A few hours passed before the doctor returned with the verdict: Charlotte indeed has epilepsy. Although I was upset by this news, I felt supported and listened to as the doctor took the time to explain everything to me in a kind and gentle way.

And life went on. Charlotte was started on Keppra, and we begin the process of scheduling follow-up appointments, including another EEG and a brain MRI. We accepted the diagnosis and tried to remain positive, but we have to admit that the shock was severe learning that our daughter was ill.

The weeks immediately following the diagnosis were difficult as Charlotte suffered from the side effects of Keppra. She had stomachache and headaches every day, and her behavior changed. She was angry, which we understood perfectly, but little by little we felt we were losing our Charlotte—creative, playful, cuddly, sporty, academic! She tired easily and became physically and verbally aggressive. Nothing interested her anymore, and she sat on the sofa without moving or speaking. She no longer wanted to dance, something she had always loved, and she didn't ever want to go out. In short, she was no longer the daughter we knew.

After two months of treatment with Keppra, I contacted the neurologist and it was decided to try a new medication for Charlotte. Goodbye Keppra, hello Micropakine. Switching from one medication to another has to be done with a progressive transition over several weeks, which was difficult for Charlotte. She experienced a lot of side effects and therefore missed a great deal of school. The tears, the slamming doors, the almost nonexistent communication, the stomachache and headaches were still sometimes there. But finally, when the transition was complete, our Charlotte resurfaced—energetic, creative, empathic, playful, mischievous, and fun. She plays with her brothers, and she hugs her father. The big cries of anger, the slamming doors, the physical and verbal confrontations disappeared.

Charlotte knows that she has epilepsy. She now will talk about it, no longer fearful to say to her teacher, "I don't feel very well." The neuropsychology tests are very positive, and her level in school is very good (she is one of the top students in the class). Charlotte knows what she must do when she feels very tired or when she has a headache.

Lately, Charlotte sometimes forgets what she wants to say; she starts a sentence and doesn't finish it, so a new EEG is going to be scheduled. As always, Charlotte's doctor is available and reassuring. Thankfully, her entire medical team is welcoming and listens; we feel we are supported.

Charlotte's diagnosis has changed our lives—in some ways for the better. Certain things that appeared to be insurmountable and serious before Charlotte was diagnosed with epilepsy now seem to be less serious. We cannot say that her epilepsy is not serious, but there is a treatment, and with diligent monitoring, everything will go well. It has helped to put things in perspective—there are worse things that can happen.

We stay positive and try to learn from it all without drama! We are parents, so anxiety is part of daily life, and more so with a sick child. But in a family with a lot of love, everything (or nearly everything) is surmountable. You learn to live with epilepsy—there is an apprehension, a fear, that does not leave us, but that we must not show. We always try to be ready, to enjoy. What more can you do?

Diana, mother of Erik, an adult, from Michigan, US

My son was inspired by his own epilepsy experience growing up.

Erik came out of the womb with an "I can do it myself" attitude. That attitude has served him well and propelled him forward through his development. He was the first of our four children and none of them came with an owner's manual. My husband and I were learning how to be parents as Erik was growing up. Who knew we would learn so much from him?

Erik was bright and energetic as a child. He read at a very early age, and I mean the newspaper, not just early reader books. When he was seven, his first-grade schoolteacher handwrote a full-page note to us saying she had some concerns and wanted us to take the details she described to his pediatrician. She detailed numerous occasions where she said Erik seemed to be daydreaming and would not respond to her when she tried to get his attention. She stated that his attention would return within a few minutes, and he would answer a question that had been asked several minutes prior as though no time had passed. We took the information seriously and saw his pediatrician, who arranged for us to see a pediatric neurologist.

I don't remember being terribly concerned after seeing the pediatrician. My mom, who cared for Erik while we worked, said, "Oh he's just like you were—a daydreamer. It's nothing." I remember thinking that I just wanted to get to the bottom of this.

My husband and I immediately liked the pediatric neurologist we were referred to. We appreciated the way he spoke directly to Erik rather than to us. But as much as we liked him, he scared us pretty quickly as he showed us what Erik's seizures looked like by simply having him breathe quickly into a paper bag (since hyperventilation would likely be a trigger for Erik's seizures). He told us Erik probably was having seizures with some frequency at school and during the night while sleeping. He asked us if Erik was a bed-wetter. He did, on occasion, wet the bed, but we always thought it was our fault for maybe not limiting fluids in the evening, so we never made a big deal of it. We just quickly changed the sheets and everyone went back to sleep.

Erik's EEG indicated a classic spike-and-wave pattern for petit mal—now called absence epilepsy. Zarontin was the first medication used, and luckily the seizures were under control with a small dose. The pediatric neurologist put our minds at ease telling us he thought Erik would outgrow the seizures and epilepsy by the onset of puberty.

All was good for a bit until, at age 10, Erik had a different seizure than his typical absence seizures. He had what looked like a grand mal seizure (now known as a generalized tonic-clonic seizure). I called the neurologist anxiously to tell him, but the doctor calmly told me he highly doubted that this was what had occurred. I remember telling him that if what had happened was not a grand mal, I never wanted to see one. He laughed and spoke to me in his calm, reassuring manner and had us bring Erik in the next day. Medication was changed to Depakote, and the neurologist reassured us that he still felt confident this would not be a lifelong issue. Again, we had good luck on a low dose. We even tried a period without medication when Erik was around age 12, which lasted for one and a half years until he started to have staring spells and a few larger seizure episodes. That resulted in him going back on Depakote.

For the next few years, Erik was a stinker. He would fake having motor seizures to get a rise out of us, and we began to ignore his antics telling him some day he would have a real seizure and we would ignore that because of all the fake ones. When Erik was 15, the neurologist took him off the Depakote as a trial prior to him becoming a driver. It did not take long before he had a seizure at home. Erik was able to get on the phone that evening with his pediatric neurologist, who agreed to some conditions that Erik wanted, while ensuring the decision would be in Erik's best interest. Erik would be allowed to remain off his medication unless he had two more seizures. Erik was of two minds: he did not want to run the risk of seizures, but he did not want to take Depakote because he didn't like how it made him feel. He opted to remain off medication and see what happened.

A second seizure occurred at home and then a third during class at school. His science teacher responded by taking the class to the library to research epilepsy while other administration tended to Erik and contacted us. I remember being so grateful for the wise science teacher, as many classmates contacted Erik that evening to inquire how he was doing. Kids can be so mean to each other in experiences like that, but

Erik never experienced bullying about his epilepsy. He was put back on medication and continued throughout the remainder of high school, and he was able to drive a car and do everything else his peers did.

Erik was inspired to pursue a career in medicine but was concerned that epilepsy would not allow him to do so. When college began, he had to change from his pediatric neurologist to an adult neurologist with whom, sadly, he was not as comfortable. Ultimately, Erik got the chance to have another trial off medication when he turned 22, and this time he didn't have any seizures. He graduated from college with a degree in electrical engineering while also taking pre-med classes and exploring how he might travel for medical volunteering. He worked as an electrical engineer for a year while preparing to write the MCAT (medical school entrance exam). He went on to an MD-PhD program while continuing to volunteer in Haiti almost every year. He survived the grueling schedule of a seven-year residency and did an extra year in fellowship for pediatric subspecialization.

Erik is now a pediatric neurosurgeon, and part of his job involves surgery for children with epilepsy. He has the heart of a servant when it comes to his patients. He understands his epilepsy surgery patients and the concern of their parents in a way that I have to believe is rare—through personal experience.

Chapter 12

Further reading and research

> Education is not the filling of a pail,
> but the lighting of a fire.
> William Butler Yeats

Further reading

For those who would like further reading on this condition, a list of recommended books, websites, and resources has been collated and will be regularly updated. Access to the list is provided in **Useful web resources.**

Research

Research serves as a cornerstone of evidence-based medicine and drives health care advancement. We discussed the importance of evidence-based medicine (or evidence-based practice) in Chapter 2. It is "the conscientious, explicit, and judicious use of current best evidence in making decisions about the care of individual patients." It combines the best available external clinical evidence from research with the clinical expertise of the professional.[83] Family priorities and preferences are also considered.[84]

Evidence is collected by carrying out scientific studies (research studies), the results of which are published as full-length, peer-reviewed research articles (or papers) in scientific journals. "Peer-reviewed" means that experts with relevant content knowledge have reviewed, challenged, and agreed that the scientific method and study conclusions based on the results are sound.

Scientific studies may also be presented in brief at conferences, and conference proceedings are often published. However, conference proceedings present preliminary results and peer review is minimal. *Therefore, full-length published research articles are the most rigorous and sound evidence.*

The above published research outputs are collectively known as scientific literature or, simply, research.

Research may also be discussed on various social media platforms such as X (formerly Twitter), Facebook, LinkedIn, and Instagram. If you consume information this way, it is always important to go back to the original source (i.e., the full-length research article) to ensure the media's portrayal of the study findings is accurate.

You may have familiarity with searching the scientific literature. If not, search engines such as PubMed (ncbi.nlm.nih.gov/pubmed) and Google Scholar (scholar.google.com) are good places to start. They provide a free abstract (a short summary of the article), which can be very useful. In the past, you generally needed to belong to an academic or medical institution to have access to full-length research articles. Many articles are now available online for free. Google Scholar provides links to many full-length articles, and some community libraries allow you to request full-length articles.

You might have heard the phrase, "Just because someone says it, doesn't mean it's true." This is worth remembering in all aspects of life, but it is also relevant to research. While research articles go through a peer review process, you should still read them with a critical eye. Ask yourself, How confident can I be in the results of this research study? Was the sample size big enough to be representative of the larger population? Did the results support the conclusion?

If you aren't a trained scientist, reviewing the quality of the evidence might be more challenging, but you can still make sure the basic methods make sense and the author's conclusions are supported by the data presented. The information below will help you learn about some research study designs and how study design affects how much confidence you can place in a study's conclusions.

Research study design

There are different research study designs, and each has its value. The quality of the evidence, or level of evidence, is graded based on the study design and how well the methods were executed. Research articles sometimes list (often in the abstract) the level of evidence from I to V, with level I being the highest.

The most common research study designs, listed from highest to lowest level of evidence, are:

- Systematic review
- Randomized controlled trial
- Cohort
- Case control
- Cross-sectional
- Case report and case series

Systematic review: A systematic review summarizes the results of several scientific studies on the same topic. They can be qualitative (descriptive) or quantitative (numerical):

- Qualitative: A summary of common themes and findings across studies but without a statistical analysis.
- Quantitative: A statistical analysis carried out that takes a weighted average of the findings across studies to produce one estimate for the effect of a treatment, for example. The quantitative approach is called a "meta-analysis."

The highest level of evidence is a systematic review of randomized controlled trials (described next), although systematic reviews can also include studies that used other types of study designs. Systematic reviews may be published by individual researchers or groups. The Cochrane collaboration is a worldwide association of researchers, health care professionals, patients, and carers that publishes systematic reviews on various topics.

Randomized controlled trial (RCT): An RCT is a study design aimed at identifying cause and effect. The cause is, for example, the treatment, and the effect is the outcome being measured. Strict control of the study method (the "C" in RCT) helps to ensure the treatment of interest is the only factor that could cause the outcome. A treatment group receives the treatment while a nontreatment group (also known as the control group) does not. The participants are randomly assigned (the "R" in RCT) to one of the groups. The random assignment is one of the key strengths of this study design because it takes care of the "unknown unknowns" that may influence the outcome. The treatment effect is found by comparing the outcomes of the treatment and nontreatment groups. RCTs are considered the highest quality study design but are still uncommon in medical literature.

Cohort: A cohort is a group of people who share a common characteristic (e.g., diagnosis, gender). In a cohort study, outcome is measured two or more times. Researchers identify the characteristic of interest and then measure the outcome, looking for associations between the two. A cohort study is a form of longitudinal study ("longitudinal" means that the same outcome is measured on the same participants two or more times over a period of time). You may come across the terms "prospective" and "retrospective" cohort studies.

- In prospective cohort studies, research questions and methods are defined, and a cohort is followed over time, collecting data.
- In retrospective cohort studies, research questions and methods are defined after data has been collected or already exists (e.g., a person's medical record).

Case control: In case control studies, researchers identify the outcome of interest, which defines the groups (e.g., infants with a specific diagnosis and typically developing infants), and then look backward in time at different factors or exposures that might have caused different outcomes. At the beginning of the study, the outcome is known, but the factors or exposures that might have caused that outcome are unknown. This is the opposite of cohort studies. Because the outcome and factors or exposures data already exist, case control studies are always retrospective.

Cross-sectional: Cross-sectional studies take measurements only once from participants. Researchers look for associations between certain factors and exposures, and outcomes.

Case report and case series: A case report (also referred to as a single-subject case study) is an account of a single patient—usually a unique case—and their medical history, status, and outcomes from a treatment, for example. A case series is a group of case reports on patients who were exposed to a similar treatment. These reports are usually retrospective, and data has already been collected by other means (usually as part of routine medical care).

Getting involved in research

There are many opportunities to become involved in research. Together with medical professionals and researchers, people with lived experience can help drive advancement in health care.

a) As a participant

Researchers working in academic and medical settings are always looking for participants for their studies. You might receive an invitation to participate in such a study via an email, letter in the mail, phone call, social media ad, or other method.

Some studies are very easy and may just involve completing one online survey; others may take more time with various measurements being taken on more than one occasion. Just as you are advised to read published research studies with a critical eye, so should you judge new research study opportunities before agreeing to participate. Participating can take time and effort—the expected time commitment will be communicated in the study recruitment material. There is often a small reimbursement offered for time spent in a study.

It's worth noting that you, as the study participant, may not personally benefit from the research study, but the collective population with the condition will likely benefit.

Clinical trials are research studies conducted to evaluate the safety and effectiveness of new medical treatments, including new medications and devices before they can be approved for widespread use. They are often conducted following a randomized controlled trial research study design.

A potential benefit of participating in clinical trials is gaining early access to new medical treatments. Even if you are assigned to the control group (which usually receives standard care), you may have early access to the new treatment once the data collection phase is complete. In addition, standard care is likely to be current best practice.

You can find information about clinical trials through various sources:

- The National Institutes of Health in the US maintains a comprehensive database, ClinicalTrials.gov, where you can learn about clinical trials around the world. You can search this database by specific medical condition, location, or other pertinent criteria to identify relevant clinical trials that may be currently enrolling participants.
- Major academic medical centers, research institutions, and hospitals often conduct clinical trials and can provide information about their ongoing studies.
- Medical professionals may be aware of ongoing clinical trials in their field and can provide guidance to families who are interested in participating.
- Organizations that support particular conditions are another source of information.

Depending on the nature of the treatment in the clinical trial, you may want to, or be required to, consult with your medical professional to help you consider the risks and benefits of participating.

b) As a co-producer

Family engagement in research (FER) plays a crucial role in fostering collaboration and helping improve study design and outcome. When families become involved in research as collaborators on a study rather than simply as participants, researchers gain valuable insights into the lived experiences and perspectives of families. Families participate at every stage of the research process: concept, design, planning, conduct, and reporting of the study findings. These opportunities are still rare but are becoming more common. As an example, a link to the FER program at Gillette Children's is included in **Useful web resources**.

The family engagement in research movement is largely attributed to the similar and earlier patient and public involvement initiative in the UK. Here are some opportunities:

- **CanChild** and the **Kids Brain Health Network** in Canada currently offer The Family Engagement in Research program, a short online training course through McMaster University Continuing Education, to train family members and researchers (including coordinators and assistants) in collaborating on research.
- Online training modules are available at **Patient-Oriented Research Curriculum in Child Health (PORCCH)**.
- The **Patient-Centered Outcomes Research Institute (PCORI)** and the **Strategy for Patient-Oriented Research (SPOR)** are two other organizations that encourage family engagement.

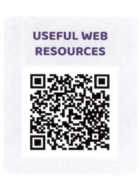

USEFUL WEB RESOURCES

Acknowledgments

> It takes a village to raise a child.
> **African proverb**

And it takes a village to produce a Healthcare Series. Publication of this series began with an idea, then with five titles, and then more titles. These acknowledgments relate to the entire series.

The formula of deep medical information interspersed with lived experience gives readers an appreciation of the childhood-acquired, often lifelong conditions. We thank the many people who contributed to each title: medical professionals at Gillette Children's who willingly came forward to lead each book; Gillette writers who did the research and writing of each; other Gillette team members who contributed from their different specialties; family authors and vignette writers who shared their personal stories; other families who shared photographs; the Gillette editing team who ensured the content and structure worked for the reader; Olwyn Roche who beautifully illustrated each title; advance readers, both professionals and families, whose feedback was invaluable; and Lina Abdennabi who coordinated Gillette Press operations. Behind every book was also a pit team who converted the finished manuscript into the book you now hold. Ruth Wilson led and looked after copyediting and proofreading. Jazmin Welch created the beautiful design and layout. Audrey McClellan indexed each title.

Smoothly creating each title required great teamwork among our villagers.

Staff at Gillette Children's provided continual support to the project and everyone involved. This included the steering committee, in particular Paula Montgomery, Dr. Micah Niermann, and Barbara Joers.

This Healthcare Series is co-published with Mac Keith Press. From the get-go, the journey with Ann-Marie Halligan and Sally Wilkinson was one of great support and collaboration.

Gillette Children's Healthcare Press

Glossary

Grasp the subject, the words will follow.
Cato the Elder

TERM	DEFINITION
Acute	Referring to something occurring with an abrupt onset.
Amplitude	The height of the *EEG wave*, which is a measure of the electric charge (i.e., the voltage) generated by the firing *neurons*.
Amygdala	A small almond-shaped structure located in the temporal lobe of the brain (in both halves) at the end of the hippocampus; responsible for processing memories and regulating emotions and behaviors (both positive and negative).
Antiseizure medication	Medication to reduce, prevent, or stop *seizures*. Also known as anticonvulsants, antiepileptic drugs (AEDs), or simply seizure medications or seizure drugs.
Artifact	An element of interference that shows up on an EEG recording due to something other than brain activity. Artifacts might be associated with eye blinks, muscle contractions, swallowing, or movement.
Atonic	Referring to the sudden loss of muscle tone in the head, trunk, jaw, and limbs.
Aura	A sensation or symptom experienced at the onset of a neurological event.
Automatisms	Repetitive, often excessive, actions involving the face, arms, or legs performed without conscious thought or intention; may include lip-smacking, chewing, repetitive hand movements, or picking at the hair or clothing.

Autonomic	Relating to involuntary actions controlled by the autonomic nervous system. In the context of a seizure, autonomic signs and symptoms may include racing heart, feelings of hot or cold, goosebumps, drooling, or gastrointestinal sensations.
Awareness	The individual's state of consciousness and knowledge of self or environment. In the context of a seizure, awareness refers to no loss of consciousness during the seizure; the individual may be able to carry on a conversation or complete a task and will likely recall the events during the seizure after it ends.
Background	Typical *baseline* brain wave activity when the brain is at rest.
Baseline	A starting point; in the context of a *seizure*, a baseline is defined as an individual's typical feelings and activities when not experiencing a seizure.
Behavioral arrest	The abrupt stopping of talking and moving; when an individual appears to "freeze up."
Benign	Referring to something that is not harmful.
Bipolar montage	In *EEG*; a common arrangement of channels organized by electrode pairs near to each other that allows for the comparison of brain areas and recognition of seizure onset zones.
Brain stem	The bottom part of the brain that connects the *cerebrum* to the spinal cord, where many functions responsible for survival are located (e.g., breathing and heart rate). The brain stem also serves as a relay station for messages between different parts of the body and the *cerebral cortex*.
Broca's area	An area of the brain involved in production of speech; located in the left (or opposite the dominant hand) frontal lobe of the brain.
Cardiac arrythmias	Atypical heart rhythms that may be too slow, too fast, or irregular.
Cardiologist	A medical professional who specializes in the care of the heart and blood vessels.

Cardiovascular conditions	Conditions that involve the heart and blood vessels.
Cardiovascular system	The system in the body made up of heart and blood vessels, including the arteries, veins, and capillaries. This system transports blood to all areas of the body.
Central nervous system (CNS)	The part of the nervous system composed of the brain and spinal cord.
Cerebral cortex	The outer layer of the *cerebrum*; made up of four lobes, it is responsible for the majority of voluntary actions, as well as thinking, learning, consciousness, personality, and many of the senses.
Cerebral palsy (CP)	A group of permanent disorders of the development of movement and posture causing activity limitation that are attributed to nonprogressive disturbances that occurred in the developing fetal or infant brain.
Cerebellum	The part of the brain located at the back of the head, under the *cerebrum*; it helps with maintaining balance and posture, coordination, and fine motor movements.
Cerebrovascular condition	A condition that involves the brain and its blood vessels.
Cerebrovascular system	A subsystem of the *cardiovascular system*; it carries blood to and from the brain.
Cerebrum	The front and upper part of the brain; the largest part of the brain. It contains an outer layer, the *cerebral cortex*, and is divided into two halves (also called hemispheres).
Channels	In *EEG*, groups of two or more electrodes capturing activity, which is reported as a single output.
Clonic	Referring to repetitive, rhythmic contractions or twitching (repeated stiffening and relaxing or jerking) of specific muscle groups of the limbs, face, or trunk.
Combined generalized and focal epilepsy	Epilepsy characterized by both *focal onset* and *generalized onset seizures*. Also called combined generalized and focal onset epilepsy.

Comorbidities	Conditions that exist along with another condition in an individual.
Corpus callosum	The communication pathway located in the center of the *cerebrum* that connects the two halves of the brain.
Déjà vu	An impression of familiarity without being able to link it to memory.
Dissociative disorder	A psychiatric condition that involves disruptions related to memory, identity, emotion, perception, and behavior.
Drug-resistant epilepsy	Epilepsy that does not achieve sustained *seizure freedom* with the use of two appropriate *antiseizure medications*. Also called drug-refractory, pharmacoresistant, or uncontrolled epilepsy.
EEG wave	In *EEG*, electrical activity in groups of *neurons*, captured by *electrodes*, and recorded on a graph.
EEG waveform	Overall shape and pattern of the *EEG waves* and how they change over time.
Electrodes	In *EEG*, small metal discs placed on the scalp (or inside the skull) that sense and record electrical activity in groups of *neurons*. Electrodes may be in the form of scalp electrodes, helmet or cap electrodes, MRI-compatible electrodes, or intracranial electrodes.
Electroencephalography (EEG)	A test that measures and records the brain's electrical activity, and generates a visual graph of brain waves. When audiovideo recording is used concurrently, it is known as VEEG (video electroencephalography).
Electrographic activity	In *EEG*, electrical activity sensed and recorded by *electrodes*.
Electrographic seizures	*Seizures* without clinical changes, but with *EEG* changes. Also called subclinical seizures.
Encephalitis	Acute inflammation of the brain tissue.
Epilepsy syndrome	A characteristic cluster of clinical and *EEG* features, often supported by specific etiological findings.

Epileptic activity	In *EEG*, abnormal electrical activity in the brain.
Epileptic seizure	A seizure associated with a diagnosis of epilepsy.
Epileptic spasm	Sudden movement that lasts for one to two seconds and involves muscle contraction causing flexion (bending), extension (straightening), or mixed flexion-extension of a limb.
Epileptiform discharges	Distinct *EEG* waveform patterns representative of epileptic activity.
Episodic dyscontrol	Recurrent attacks of uncontrollable rage and violence followed by exhaustion and difficulty recalling the event. Also called intermittent explosive disorder.
Etiology	The cause of a condition.
Febrile seizure	A *provoked seizure* that occurs in an infant or child between six months and five years of age; associated with a temperature of at least 100.4 °F (38 °C), and without brain or spinal cord infection.
Focal epilepsy	Epilepsy characterized by *focal onset seizures*. Also called focal onset epilepsy.
Focal onset seizure	A *seizure* that starts from one half of the brain and leads to signs and symptoms on one side of the body (opposite to the half of the brain in which the seizure occurs). These are often referred to as focal seizures.
Frequency	A measurement of how many *EEG waves* occur per second.
Gastroenteritis	A condition that causes inflammation and irritation of the digestive tract, leading to vomiting, diarrhea, or nausea.
Gastroenterologist	A medical professional who specializes in the care of the digestive system, including the stomach and intestines.
Gastroesophageal reflux disease (GERD)	A condition where liquid contents from the stomach go back into the esophagus. Also called acid reflux.
Gene	The basic unit of heredity transferred from parent to offspring.

Generalized epilepsy	Epilepsy characterized by *generalized onset seizures*. Also called generalized onset epilepsy.
Generalized onset seizure	A *seizure* that starts from both halves of the brain and leads to signs and symptoms on both sides of the body; often referred to as a generalized seizure.
Genetic epilepsy	Epilepsy caused by or closely associated with pathologic changes in *genes*.
Genetics	A branch of science that studies genes or heredity.
Hippocampus	An area of the brain located deep within the temporal lobe (on both halves of the brain), primarily associated with memory, particularly long-term memory storage and consolidation and decision-making.
Hydrocephalus	A condition in which there is a buildup of cerebrospinal fluid (fluid that surrounds the brain and spinal canal) in cavities (ventricles) in the brain.
Hyperkinetic	Referring to excessive, abnormal, and large involuntary movements that may include motions such as thrashing or leg pedaling.
Hypoglycemia	A condition with lower than typical blood glucose (sugar) levels, resulting in confusion, a loss of or decrease in consciousness, lack of coordination, difficulties with speech, and tremors.
Ictal phase	The active phase of a *seizure*.
Immune epilepsy	Epilepsy caused by an alteration in the body's defense system against infections.
Impaired awareness	Alteration or loss of consciousness during a *seizure*; the individual may appear confused, may not be able to respond, or may experience a loss of consciousness and will typically not fully recall the events of the seizure after it ends.
Infectious epilepsy	Epilepsy caused by a previous (not *acute*) infection in the brain.
Infertility	The failure to achieve a pregnancy after 12 months or more of regular, unprotected sexual intercourse.

International 10–20 system	A commonly used pattern of electrode placement; electrodes are placed either 10 or 20 percent of the total distance of bony landmarks on the skull.
Ions	Charged particles; examples include sodium, potassium, chloride.
Ketogenic diet	A form of dietary therapy that restricts the intake of carbohydrates, allows for a moderate amount of protein, and greatly increases the intake of fats to induce a metabolic state known as ketosis in the individual.
Meningitis	Acute inflammation of the membranes (meninges) surrounding the brain and spinal cord.
Metabolic	Referring to chemical processes that allow cells in the body to convert food into energy.
Metabolic epilepsy	Epilepsy caused by a *metabolic* disorder.
Migraine	A type of headache with moderate to severe throbbing and pulsating pain.
Monotherapy	The use of one *antiseizure medication*.
Motor cortex	The area of the *cerebral cortex* in the frontal lobe responsible for voluntary movements.
Motor signs	Uncontrolled physical movement experienced by the individual during the *seizure* that can be seen by observers.
Myoclonic	Single or multiple involuntary muscle contractions that are sudden and last less than a second.
Narcolepsy	A disorder characterized by excessive sleepiness during the day and often presenting with irresistible sleep attacks.
Neuromodulation	Repetitive electrical discharges administered through a device for the management of epilepsy; these devices are surgically implanted.
Neuron	The smallest unit of the nervous system; electrically excitable cells that carry information (signals) between the *central nervous system* and the rest of the body as electrical impulses.

Neurotransmitters	Special chemicals that carry a signal across the *synapse* either stimulating (exciting) the next *neuron* or cell to take action or preventing (inhibiting) it from doing so.
Nonmotor signs and symptoms	What the individual who is seizing experiences; these may be observed by others if they include a lack of movement, emotional outbursts, or a change in vital signs.
Parasomnias	A group of sleep disorders characterized by unusual behaviors that occur just prior to falling asleep, while asleep, or just upon waking up and may be accompanied by loss of consciousness and the inability to recall the event.
Phase	In *EEG*, a measurement of the timing relationship between different *EEG waves*.
Polytherapy	The use of more than one *antiseizure medication*.
Postictal phase	The last stage of a *seizure*.
Postural orthostatic tachycardia syndrome (POTS)	A group of conditions where bloodflow to the heart is impacted after an individual changes position, resulting in a symptom known as orthostatic intolerance. Individuals with orthostatic intolerance feel faint or lightheaded when moving from lying to standing.
Preictal phase	The first stage of a *seizure*.
Prevalence	The proportion of a population with a specific characteristic, or condition, in a specified period, often expressed as a percentage.
Prognosis	The prospect of recovering from injury or disease, or a prediction or forecast of the course and outcome of a medical condition.
Provoked seizure	A *seizure* associated with a *systemic* injury or a brain injury. Also called an acute symptomatic seizure.
Psychogenic nonepileptic seizures (PNES)	Involuntary events that may last for several minutes (sometimes 15 to 30 minutes or longer) and often involve loss of consciousness or motor signs such as irregular jerking or shaking of the limbs and falling.

Reflex seizure	A type of *provoked seizure* that occurs after a particular stimulus; very rare, and is typically associated with an *epilepsy syndrome* (e.g., reading epilepsy and startle epilepsy).
Remission	Referring to a state where an individual with epilepsy is seizure-free for at least six months.
Resolved	Referring to a state where an individual with epilepsy has remained seizure-free for 10 years, with no *antiseizure medications* for the last 5 years, or the individual had an age-dependent *epilepsy syndrome* and is now past the applicable age for this diagnosis (i.e., self-limited neonatal or infantile epilepsy syndromes).
Risk factor	An aspect of personal behavior or lifestyle, an environmental exposure, or an inborn or inherited characteristic associated with an increased occurrence of disease or other health-related event or condition.
Seizure	Uncontrolled, abnormal electrical activity of the brain that may cause changes in the level of consciousness, behavior, memory, or feelings.
Seizure freedom	A set period without any *seizures*.
Seizure mimic	An event that appears to be a *seizure* but is not; rather, it is due to another condition. called nonepilpetic event.
Seizure threshold	The point at which an individual's brain is likely to experience a *seizure*; the theoretical sum of the various triggers that are likely enough for the abnormal electrical activity to initiate a seizure.
Self-limiting	Referring to a disease or condition that spontaneously resolves.
Shunt	A device inserted into the ventricles of the brain; the shunt tubing (catheter) drains the cerebrospinal fluid from the ventricles and transports it to a reservoir where it is stored and then pumped to the peritoneal cavity (a space within the abdominal area not occupied by the abdominal organs). There, the fluid is absorbed by the body.

Sleep myoclonus	A sudden, involuntary muscle jerk often accompanied by a hallucination of movement, experienced as a feeling of falling. These events are very brief and occur during sleep transitions (falling asleep or waking up).
Somatosensory cortex	The area of the *cerebral cortex* in the parietal lobe responsible for receiving sensory information.
Spasm	A brief, involuntary muscle contraction.
Status epilepticus	A life-threatening condition in which *seizures* last more than five minutes or occur in close succession (one after the other, without a return to *baseline*).
Stereotypies	Semivoluntary repetitive movements that are often rhythmic and may include clapping or arm shaking.
Stroke	A condition in which a blood vessel in the brain is either blocked or ruptured, damaging the brain and causing symptoms such as paralysis, speech problems, and memory loss.
Structural epilepsy	Epilepsy caused by a distinct abnormality of the brain.
Subclinical seizure	*Seizures* without clinical changes but with *EEG* changes. Also called *electrographic seizures*.
Sudden unexpected death in epilepsy (SUDEP)	The death of an individual with epilepsy when no other cause of death can be found.
Synapse	The junction between the sending neuron and the receiving neuron or cell.
Syncope	A condition that involves *self-limiting* transient (temporary) loss of consciousness with the inability to maintain a standing or unsupported posture and may be accompanied by brief jerking movements. Also called fainting spell.
Systemic	Referring to affecting the entire body.
Tic	An involuntary, sudden, rapid, and repetitive sound or movement.
Tonic	Referring to a sustained muscle contraction resulting in a sudden stiffness or tense posture; typically seen as an extension of the limb.

Tonic-clonic	Referring to movements that occur in two stages: tonic movements in which the individual loses consciousness and the muscles suddenly contract (lasting about 10 to 20 seconds) followed immediately by clonic movements in which the muscles repetitively and rhythmically contract (lasting 1 or 2 minutes or less).
Transient ischemic attack (TIA)	A condition in which a blood vessel in the brain is temporarily (transient; lasting for a short time) blocked causing temporary symptoms like a *stroke*.
Unknown epilepsy	Epilepsy without a definitive cause.
Unknown onset seizure	A *seizure* with an unclear starting location in the brain.
Unprovoked seizure	A *seizure* that occurs without a specific *acute* cause.
Wernicke's area	An area of the brain located in the left (or opposite the dominant hand) temporal lobe; involved in understanding and comprehension of speech.

References

1. World Health Organization (2001) *International Classification of Functioning, Disability and Health (ICF)*. [online] Available at: <https://www.who.int/standards/classifications/international-classification-of-functioning-disability-and-health> [Accessed February 22 2024].
2. Huff JS, Murr N (2023) *Seizure*. [e-book] Treasure Island, StatPearls Publishing. Available at: National Library of Medicine <https://www.ncbi.nlm.nih.gov/books/NBK430765/> [Accessed February 9 2024].
3. Kiriakopoulos E (2019) *Understanding Seizures*. [online] Available at: <https://www.epilepsy.com/what-is-epilepsy/understanding-seizures> [Accessed February 9 2024].
4. Epilepsy Foundation (2024) *What is epilepsy?* [online] Available at: <https://www.epilepsy.com/what-is-epilepsy> [Accessed September 25 2024].
5. Fisher RS, Acevedo C, Arzimanoglou A, et al. (2014) ILAE official report: A practical clinical definition of epilepsy. *Epilepsia*, 55, 475–482.
6. International League Against Epilepsy (2014) *Definition of Epilepsy 2014*. [online] Available at: <https://www.ilae.org/guidelines/definition-and-classification/definition-of-epilepsy-2014> [Accessed March 4 2024].
7. Wirrell EC, Nabbout R, Scheffer IE, et al. (2022) Methodology for classification and definition of epilepsy syndromes with list of syndromes: Report of the ILAE Task Force on Nosology and Definitions. *Epilepsia*, 63, 1333–1348.
8. Joshi C (2019) *Reflex epilepsies*. [online] Available at: <https://www.epilepsy.com/what-is-epilepsy/syndromes/reflex-epilepsies#What-is-meant-by-reflex-epilepsy?> [Accessed September 25 2024].
9. Eilbert W, Chan C (2022) Febrile seizures: A review. *J Am Coll Emerg Physicians Open*, 3, 1–6.
10. Sawires R, Buttery J, Fahey M (2021) A review of febrile seizures: Recent advances in understanding of febrile seizure pathophysiology and commonly implicated viral triggers. *Front Pediatr*, 9, 1–8.
11. Cullen C (2022) *Pediatric febrile and first-time seizures*, [online] Available at: <https://www.reliasmedia.com/articles/149531-pediatric-febrile-and-first-time-seizures> [Accessed September 13 2024].
12. Fisher RS, Cross JH, French JA, et al. (2017) Operational classification of seizure types by the International League Against Epilepsy: Position paper of the ILAE Commission for Classification and Terminology. *Epilepsia*, 58, 522–530.
13. Merriam-Webster (2024) *Convulsion*. [online] Available at: <https://www.merriam-webster.com/dictionary/convulsion> [Accessed September 13 2024].

14. Gobbi G, Mainardi P, Striano P, Preda A (2019) Epilepsy, coeliac disease and other inflammatory bowel diseases. In: Mula M, ed., *The Comorbidities of Epilepsy*. London: Academic Press, pp 107–130.
15. Scheffer IE, Berkovic S, Capovilla G, et al. (2017) ILAE classification of the epilepsies: Position paper of the ILAE Commission for Classification and Terminology. *Epilepsia*, 58, 512–521.
16. National Human Genome Research Institute (2024) *Talking glossary of genomic and genetic terms*. [online] Available at: <https://www.genome.gov/genetics-glossary> [Accessed September 20 2024].
17. Centers for Disease Control and Prevention (2024) *Epidemiology Glossary*. [online] Available at: <https://www.cdc.gov/reproductive-health/glossary/> [Accessed June 24 2024].
18. Schachter SC (2024) *What are the risk factors of seizures?* [online] Available at: <https://www.epilepsy.com/what-is-epilepsy/understanding-seizures/risk-factors> [Accessed 2024 September 13].
19. Epilepsy Foundation (2022) *Who can get epilepsy?* [online] Available at: <https://www.epilepsy.com/what-is-epilepsy/understanding-seizures/who-gets-epilepsy> [Accessed September 13 2024].
20. Tenny S (2023) *Prevalence*. [online] Available at: <https://www.statpearls.com/articlelibrary/viewarticle/27708/> [Accessed September 13 2024].
21. World Health Organization (2019) Epilepsy a public health imperative [pdf], Geneva. Available at: <https://www.who.int/publications/i/item/epilepsy-a-public-health-imperative> [Accessed September 13 2024].
22. Falco-Walter J (2020) Epilepsy-definition, classification, pathophysiology, and epidemiology. *Semin Neurol*, 40, 617–623.
23. Beghi E (2020) The epidemiology of epilepsy. *Neuroepidemiology*, 54, 185-191.
24. World Health Organization (2024) *Epilepsy*. [online] Available at: <https://www.who.int/news-room/fact-sheets/detail/epilepsy> [Accessed September 13 2024].
25. Biset G, Abebaw N, Gebeyehu NA, et al. (2024) Prevalence, incidence, and trends of epilepsy among children and adolescents in Africa: A systematic review and meta-analysis. *BMC Public Health*, 24, 1–14.
26. Epilepsy Foundation (2020) *Seizure first aid resources*. [online] Available at: <https://www.epilepsy.com/tools-resources/forms-resources/first-aid> [Accessed September 13 2024].
27. World Health Organization (2024) *Newborn Health*. [online] Available at: <https://www.who.int/westernpacific/health-topics/newborn-health> [Accessed 2024 September 13].
28. Centers for Disease Control and Prevention (2024) *Positive parenting tips: Infants (0–1 years)*. [online] Available at: <https://www.cdc.gov/child-development/positive-parenting-tips/infants.html> [Accessed September 25 2024].
29. National Institute of Diabetes and Digestive and Kidney Diseases (2020) *Definition and facts for GER and GERD* [online] Available at: <https://www.niddk.nih.gov/health-information/digestive-diseases/acid-reflux-ger-gerd-adults/definition-facts> [Accessed September 13 2024].

30. Bayram AK, Canpolat M, Karacabey N, et al. (2016) Misdiagnosis of gastroesophageal reflux disease as epileptic seizures in children. *Brain and Development*, 38, 274–279.
31. Stainman RS, Kossoff EH (2020) Seizure mimics in children: An age-based approach. *Curr Probl Pediatr Adolesc Health Care*, 50, 1–11.
32. Fine A, Wirrell EC (2020) Seizures in children. *Pediatr Rev*, 41, 321–347.
33. Patil S, Tas. V (2023) *Sandifer Syndrome*. [e-book] Treasure Island, StatPearls. Available at: National Library of Medicine <https://www.ncbi.nlm.nih.gov/books/NBK558906/> [Accessed September 13 2024].
34. Goldman RD (2015) Breath-holding spells in infants. *Can Fam Physician*, 61, 149–150.
35. Ghossein J, Pohl D (2019) Benign spasms of infancy: a mimicker of infantile epileptic disorders. *Epileptic Disord*, 21, 585–589.
36. National Institute of Diabetes and Digestive and Kidney Diseases (2021) *Low blood glucose (hypoglycemia)*. [online] Available at: <https://www.niddk.nih.gov/health-information/diabetes/overview/preventing-problems/low-blood-glucose-hypoglycemia#whatis> [Accessed September 2024].
37. Malmgren K, Reuber M, Appleton R (2012) Differential diagnosis of epilepsy. In: Shorvon S, Guerrini R, Cook M, Lhatoo S, eds., *Oxford Textbook of Epilepsy and Epileptic Seizures*. Oxford: Oxford University Press, pp 81–94.
38. National Institute of Neurological Disorders and Stroke (2024) *Migraine*. [online] Available at: <https://www.ninds.nih.gov/health-information/disorders/migraine> [Accessed 2024 September 13].
39. Babiker MO, Prasad M (2015) Fifteen-minute consultation: When is a seizure not a seizure? Part 2, the older child. *Arch Dis Child Educ Pract Ed*, 100, 295–300.
40. Charles A (2018) The migraine aura. *Continuum*, 24, 1009–1022.
41. Leibetseder A, Eisermann M, LaFrance WCJ, Nobili L, Von Oertzen TJ (2020) How to distinguish seizures from non-epileptic manifestations. *Epileptic Disord*, 22, 716–738.
42. Ueda K, Black KJ (2021) A comprehensive review of tic disorders in children. *J Clin Med*, 10, 1–32.
43. National Institute of Neurological Disorders and Stroke (2024) *Narcolepsy*. [online] Available at: <https://www.ninds.nih.gov/health-information/disorders/narcolepsy#toc-what-is-narcolepsy-> [Accessed September 13 2024].
44. Benbadis S (2009) The differential diagnosis of epilepsy: A critical review. *Epilepsy Behav*, 15, 15–21.
45. Derry CP (2014) Sleeping in fits and starts: A practical guide to distinguishing nocturnal epilepsy from sleep disorders. *Pract Neurol*, 14, 391–398.
46. Singh S, Kaur H, Singh S, Khawaja I (2018) Parasomnias: A comprehensive review. *Cureus*, 10, 1–9.
47. National Institute of Neurological Disorders and Stroke (2024) *Myoclonus*. [online] Available at: <https://www.ninds.nih.gov/health-information/disorders/myoclonus> [Accessed 2024 September 13].
48. Wirrell E (2021) *Imitators of epilepsy*. [online] Available at: <https://www.epilepsy.com/diagnosis/imitators-epilepsy> [Accessed September 13 2024].

49. World Health Organization (2024) *Adolescent Health.* [online] Available at: <https://www.who.int/health-topics/adolescent-health> [Accessed September 13 2024].
50. American Psychiatric Association (2022) *What are dissociative disorders?* [online] Available at: <https://www.psychiatry.org/patients-families/dissociative-disorders/what-are-dissociative-disorders> [Accessed September 13 2024].
51. McTague A, Appleton R (2010) Episodic dyscontrol syndrome. *Arch Dis Child,* 95, 841–842.
52. Cho Y (2016) Management of patients with long QT syndrome. *Korean Circ J,* 46, 747–752.
53. National Institute of Neurological Disorders and Stroke (2024) *Postural tachycardia syndrome (POTS).* [online] Available at: <https://www.ninds.nih.gov/health-information/disorders/postural-tachycardia-syndrome-pots> [Accessed September 13 2024].
54. American Stroke Association (2024) *Effects of stroke.* [online] Available at: <https://www.stroke.org/en/about-stroke/effects-of-stroke> [Accessed September 13 2024].
55. American Stroke Association (2024) *Transient ischemic attack (TIA).* [online] Available at: <https://www.stroke.org/en/about-stroke/types-of-stroke/tia-transient-ischemic-attack> [Accessed September 13 2024].
56. Huff JS, Lui F, Murr NI (2024) *Psychogenic Nonepileptic Seizures.* [e-book] Treasure Island (FL), StatPearls. Available at: National Library of Medicine <https://www.ncbi.nlm.nih.gov/books/NBK441871/> [Accessed September 13 2024].
57. Winton-Brown T, Wilson SJ, Felmingham K, et al. (2023) Principles for delivering improved care of people with functional seizures: Closing the treatment gap. *Aust N Z J Psychiatry,* 57, 1511–1517.
58. Merriam-Webster (2024) *Self-limiting.* [online] Available at: <https://www.merriam-webster.com/dictionary/self-limiting> [Accessed September 13 2024].
59. Taşdelen A, Arzu E (2022) Transient loss of consciousness in children: Syncope or epileptic seizure? *Neurol Asia,* 27, 309–315.
60. Yeom JS, Woo HO (2023) Pediatric syncope: Pearls and pitfalls in history taking. *Clin Exp Pediatr,* 66, 88–97.
61. Wolf P, Benbadis S, Dimova PS, et al. (2020) The importance of semiological information based on epileptic seizure history. *Epileptic Disord,* 22, 15–31.
62. Beniczky S, Tatum WO, Blumenfeld H, et al. (2022) Seizure semiology: ILAE glossary of terms and their significance. *Epileptic Disord,* 24, 447–495.
63. Surges R, Shmuely S, Dietze C, Ryvlin P, Thijs RD (2021) Identifying patients with epilepsy at high risk of cardiac death: Signs, risk factors and initial management of high risk of cardiac death. *Epileptic Disord,* 23, 17–39.
64. Bayard M, Gerayli F, Holt J (2023) Syncope: Evaluation and differential diagnosis. *Am Fam Physician,* 108, 454–463.
65. Pohlmann-Eden B, Beghi E, Camfield C, Camfield P (2006) The first seizure and its management in adults and children. *BMJ,* 332, 339–342.

66. Beghi E, Giussani G, Sander JW (2015) The natural history and prognosis of epilepsy. *Epileptic Disord*, 17, 243–253.
67. Kiriakopoulos E (2024) *Types of seizures*. [online] Available at: <https://www.epilepsy.com/what-is-epilepsy/seizure-types> [Accessed September 16 2024].
68. Piña-Garza JE, James KC (2019) Paroxysmal disorders. In: Piña-Garza JE, James KC, eds., *Fenichel's Clinical Pediatric Neurology*. 8th ed. Philadelphia: Elsevier, pp 1–48.
69. Kiriakopoulos E (2022) *Focal impaired awareness seizures (Complex Partial Seizures)*. [online] Available at: <https://www.epilepsy.com/what-is-epilepsy/seizure-types/focal-onset-impaired-awareness-seizures> [Accessed September 13 2024].
70. Gillette Children's (2024) *Epilepsy and seizures*. [online] Available at: <https://www.gillettechildrens.org/conditions-care/epilepsy-and-seizures/epilepsy-symptoms> [Accessed September 13 2024].
71. Kiriakopoulos E (2024) *Clonic seizures*. [online] Available at: <https://www.epilepsy.com/what-is-epilepsy/seizure-types/clonic-seizures#What-is-a-clonic-seizure?> [Accessed September 13 2024].
72. Kiriakopoulos E, Osborne Shafer P (2017) *Tonic seizures*. [online] Available at: <https://www.epilepsy.com/what-is-epilepsy/seizure-types/tonic-seizures> [Accessed September 13 2024].
73. Merriam-Webster (2024) *Aura*. [online] Available at: <https://www.merriam-webster.com/dictionary/auras> [Accessed September 2024].
74. Schachter SC (2022) *What happens during a seizure?* [online] Available at: <https://www.epilepsy.com/what-is-epilepsy/understanding-seizures/what-happens-during-seizure> [Accessed September 13 2024].
75. Waxenbaum JA, Reddy V, Varacallo M (2023) *Anatomy, Autonomic Nervous System*. [e-book] Treasure Island (FL), StatPearls. Available at: National Library of Medicine <https://www.ncbi.nlm.nih.gov/books/NBK539845/> [Accessed September 16 2024].
76. National Center for Complementary and Integrative Health (2024) *4 Fast facts about the somatosensory system*. [online] Available at: <https://www.nccih.nih.gov/health/4-fast-facts-about-the-somatosensory-system> [Accessed September 16 2024].
77. Hernandez A, Joshi C (2019) *Epilepsy myoclonic absences*. [online] Available at: <https://www.epilepsy.com/what-is-epilepsy/syndromes/epilepsy-myoclonic-absences> [Accessed September 16 2024].
78. Hernandez A, Wirrell E (2019) *Epilepsy eyelid myoclonia Jeavons syndrome*. [online] Available at: <https://www.epilepsy.com/what-is-epilepsy/syndromes/epilepsy-eyelid-myoclonia-jeavons-syndrome> [Accessed September 16 2024].
79. Kiriakopoulos E (2024) *Focal bilateral tonic clonic seizures (secondarily generalized seizures)*. [online] Available at: <https://www.epilepsy.com/what-is-epilepsy/seizure-types/focal-bilateral-tonic-clonic-seizures#What-is-a-focal-to-bilateral-tonic-clonic-seizure-(secondarily-generalized-seizure)?> [Accessed September 16 2024].
80. Pottkämper JCM, Hofmeijer J, Van Waarde JA, Van Putten M (2020) The postictal state—What do we know? *Epilepsia*, 61, 1045–1061.

81. Nascimento FA, Friedman D, Peters JM, et al. (2023) Focal epilepsies: Update on diagnosis and classification. *Epileptic Disord*, 25, 1–17.
82. Nickels KC, Zaccariello MJ, Hamiwka LD, Wirrell EC (2016) Cognitive and neurodevelopmental comorbidities in paediatric epilepsy. *Nat Rev Neurol*, 12, 465–476.
83. International League Against Epilepsy (2024) *Definition & classification*. [online] Available at: <https://www.ilae.org/guidelines/definition-and-classification> [Accessed September 16 2024].
84. CanChild (2024) *Family-Centred Service*. [online] Available at: <https://canchild.ca/en/research-in-practice/family-centred-service> [Accessed February 22 2024].
85. Sackett DL, Rosenberg WM, Gray JA, Haynes RB, Richardson WS (1996) Evidence based medicine: What it is and what it isn't. *BMJ*, 312, 71–2.
86. Siminoff LA (2013) Incorporating patient and family preferences into evidence-based medicine. *BMC Med Inform Decis Mak*, 13, 1–7.
87. Agency for Healthcare Research and Quality (2020) The SHARE Approach: A Model for Shared Decisionmaking—Fact Sheet, Available at: <https://www.ahrq.gov/health-literacy/professional-training/shared-decision/tools/factsheet.html> [Accessed February 18 2024].
88. International League Against Epilepsy (2024) *SUDEP (Sudden Unexpected Death in Epilepsy)*. [online] Available at: <https://www.ilae.org/patient-care/sudep/sudep-sudden-unexpected-death-in-epilepsy> [Accessed September 16 2024].
89. Whitney R, Sharma S, Ramachandrannair R (2023) Sudden unexpected death in epilepsy in children. *Dev Med Child Neurol*, 65, 1150–1156.
90. Centers for Disease Control and Prevention (2024) *Sudden unexpected death in epilepsy*. [online] Available at: <https://www.cdc.gov/epilepsy/sudep/index.html> [Accessed September 25 2024].
91. Thau L, Reddy V, Singh P (2022) *Anatomy, Central Nervous System*. [e-book] Treasure Island (FL), StatPearls. Available at: National Library of Medicine <https://www.ncbi.nlm.nih.gov/books/NBK542179/> [Accessed September 16 2024].
92. Jimsheleishvili S, Dididze M (2023) *Neuroanatomy, Cerebellum*. [e-book] Treasure Island (FL), StatPearls. Available at: National Library of Medicine <www.ncbi.nlm.nih.gov/books/NBK538167/> [Accessed September 25 2024].
93. Netter FH (2023) *Netter Atlas of Human Anatomy: Classic regional approach*. New York: Elsevier.
94. Kumar A, Ighodaro ET, Sharma S (2024) *Focal Impaired Awareness Seizure*. [e-book] Treasure Island (FL), StatPearls. Available at: National Library of Medicine <https://www.ncbi.nlm.nih.gov/books/NBK519030/> [Accessed September 16 2024].
95. Chowdhury FA, Silva R, Whatley B, Walker MC (2021) Localisation in focal epilepsy: A practical guide. *Pract Neurol*, 21, 481–491.
96. Stinnett TJ, Reddy V, Zabel MK (2023) *Neuroanatomy, Broca Area*. [e-book] Treasure Island (FL), StatPearls. Available at: National Library of Medicine <https://www.ncbi.nlm.nih.gov/books/NBK526096/> [Accessed September 18 2023].

97. Javed K, Reddy V, Das JM, Wroten M (2023) *Neuroanatomy, Wernicke Area.* [e-book] Treasure Island (FL), StatPearls. Available at: National Library of Medicine <https://www.ncbi.nlm.nih.gov/books/NBK533001/> [Accessed September 20 2024].
98. Acharya AB, Wroten M (2023) *Broca Aphasia.* [e-book] Treasure Island (FL), StatPearls. Available at: National Library of Medicine <https://www.ncbi.nlm.nih.gov/books/NBK436010/> [Accessed September 20 2024].
99. Fogwe LA, Reddy V, Mesfin FB (2023) *Neuroanatomy, Hippocampus.* [e-book] Treasure Island (FL), StatPearls. Available at: National Library of Medicine <https://www.ncbi.nlm.nih.gov/books/NBK482171/> [Accessed September 20 2024].
100. Epilepsy Foundation (2014) *Thinking and memory.* [online] Available at: <https://www.epilepsy.com/complications-risks/thinking-and-memory> [Accessed September 20 2024].
101. Walker MC (2015) Hippocampal sclerosis: Causes and prevention. *Semin Neurol*, 35, 193–200.
102. Abuhasan Q, Reddy V, Siddiqui W (2023) *Neuroanatomy, Amygdala.* [e-book] Treasure Island (FL), StatPearls. Available at: National Library of Medicine <https://www.ncbi.nlm.nih.gov/books/NBK537102/> [Accessed September 20 2024].
103. Vinti V, Dell'Isola GB, Tascini G, et al. (2021) Temporal lobe epilepsy and psychiatric comorbidity. *Front Neurol*, 12, 1–8.
104. Ludwig PE, Reddy V, Varacallo M (2023) *Neuroanatomy, Neurons.* [e-book] Treasure Island (FL), StatPearls. Available at: National Library of Medicine <https://www.ncbi.nlm.nih.gov/books/NBK441977/> [Accessed September 20 2024].
105. Schachter SC (2024) *Seizure triggers.* [online] Available at: <https://www.epilepsy.com/what-is-epilepsy/seizure-triggers> [Accessed September 20 2024].
106. Benbadis SR, Beniczky S, Bertram E, MacIver S, Moshé SL (2020) The role of EEG in patients with suspected epilepsy. *Epileptic Disord*, 22, 143–155.
107. Nobili L, Frauscher B, Eriksson S, et al. (2022) Sleep and epilepsy: A snapshot of knowledge and future research lines. *J Sleep Res*, 31, 1–11.
108. Tatum WO, Husain AM, Benbadis SR, Kaplan PW (2008) *Handbook of EEG Interpretation.* New York: Demos Medical Publishing, LLC.
109. Britton JW, Frey LC, Hopp JL, et al. (2016) *Electroencephalography.* Chicago: American Epilepsy Society.
110. Arbune AA, Conradsen I, Cardenas DP, et al. (2020) Ictal quantitative surface electromyography correlates with postictal EEG suppression. *Neurology*, 94, 2567–2576.
111. Beniczky S, Conradsen I, Moldovan M, et al. (2014) Quantitative analysis of surface electromyography during epileptic and nonepileptic convulsive seizures. *Epilepsia*, 55, 1128–1134.
112. Kane N, Acharya J, Benickzy S, et al. (2017) A revised glossary of terms most commonly used by clinical electroencephalographers and updated proposal for the report format of the EEG findings. Revision 2017. *Clin Neurophysiol Pract*, 2, 170–185.

113. Sirven JI, Devinsky O (2013) *Interictal problems.* [online] Available at: <https://www.epilepsy.com/complications-risks/moods-behavior/interictal-problems> [Accessed September 20 2024].
114. Drane DL, Ojemann JG, Kim MS, et al. (2016) Interictal epileptiform discharge effects on neuropsychological assessment and epilepsy surgical planning. *Epilepsy Behav,* 56, 131–138.
115. Smith MS, Matthews R, Rajnik M, Mukherji P (2024) *Infantile Epileptic Spasms Syndrome (West Syndrome).* [e-book] Treasure Island (FL), StatPearls. Available at: National Library of Medicine <https://www.ncbi.nlm.nih.gov/books/NBK537251/> [Accessed September 25 2024].
116. Bruno E, Viana PF, Sperling MR, Richardson MP (2020) Seizure detection at home: Do devices on the market match the needs of people living with epilepsy and their caregivers? *Epilepsia,* 61 Suppl 1, 11–24.
117. Beniczky S, Wiebe S, Jeppesen J, et al. (2021) Automated seizure detection using wearable devices: A clinical practice guideline of the International League Against Epilepsy and the International Federation of Clinical Neurophysiology. *Clin Neurophysiol,* 132, 1173–1184.
118. Raju H, Sharma A, Smeaton A, Smeaton A (2023) Automatic detection of signalling behaviour from assistance dogs as they forecast the onset of epileptic seizures in humans. In: *Proceedings of the 38th ACM/SIGAPP Symposium on Applied Computing,* Tallinn, Estonia 2023, New York, Association for Computing Machinery.
119. Epilepsy Foundation (2007) *Seizure-alert dogs: Just the facts, hold the media hype.* [online] Available at: <https://www.epilepsy.com/stories/seizure-alert-dogs-just-facts-hold-media-hype> [Accessed September 20 2024].
120. Kirton A, Winter A, Wirrell E, Snead OC (2008) Seizure response dogs: Evaluation of a formal training program. *Epilepsy Behav,* 13, 499–504.
121. Catala A, Grandgeorge M, Schaff JL, et al. (2019) Dogs demonstrate the existence of an epileptic seizure odour in humans. *Sci Rep,* 9, 1–7.
122. Maa E, Arnold J, Ninedorf K, Olsen H (2021) Canine detection of volatile organic compounds unique to human epileptic seizure. *Epilepsy Behav,* 115, 1–8.
123. Martos Martinez-Caja A, De Herdt V, Boon P, et al. (2019) Seizure-alerting behavior in dogs owned by people experiencing seizures. *Epilepsy Behav,* 94, 104–111.
124. Shaikh Z, Torres A, Takeoka M (2019) Neuroimaging in pediatric epilepsy. *Brain Sci,* 9, 1–14.
125. Wang YQ, Wen Y, Wang MM, Zhang YW, Fang ZX (2021) Prolactin levels as a criterion to differentiate between psychogenic non-epileptic seizures and epileptic seizures: A systematic review. *Epilepsy Res,* 169, 1–10.
126. Nardone R, Brigo F, Trinka E (2016) Acute symptomatic seizures caused by electrolyte disturbances. *J Clin Neurol,* 12, 21–33.
127. Panayiotopoulos CP (2005) Clinical aspects of the diagnosis of epileptic seizures and epileptic syndromes. In: Panayiotopoulos CP, ed., *The Epilepsies: Seizures, syndromes and management.* Oxfordshire (UK): Bladon Medical Publishing.

128. Sánchez López De Nava A, Raja A (2024) *Physiology, Metabolism.* [e-book] Treasure Island (FL), StatPearls. Available at: National Library of Medicine <https://www.ncbi.nlm.nih.gov/books/NBK546690/>.
129. Lewis T, Stone WL (2024) *Biochemistry, Proteins Enzymes.* [e-book] Treasure Island (FL), StatPearls. Available at: National Library of Medicine <https://pubmed.ncbi.nlm.nih.gov/32119368/> [Accessed September 20 2024].
130. Mukherji P, Azhar Y, Sharma S (2023) *Toxicology Screening.* [e-book] Treasure Island (FL), StatPearls. Available at: National Library of Medicine <https://www.ncbi.nlm.nih.gov/books/NBK499901/> [Accessed September 20 2023].
131. Balestrini S, Arzimanoglou A, Blümcke I, et al. (2021) The aetiologies of epilepsy. *Epileptic Disord,* 23, 1–16.
132. Centers for Disease Control and Prevention (2024) *Genetic testing.* [online] Available at: <https://www.cdc.gov/genomics-and-health/about/genetic-testing.html> [Accessed September 20 2024].
133. MedlinePlus (2023) *Etiology.* [online] Available at: <https://medlineplus.gov/ency/article/002356.htm> [Accessed September 20 2024].
134. Patel P, Moshé SL (2020) The evolution of the concepts of seizures and epilepsy: What's in a name? *Epilepsia Open,* 5, 22–35.
135. Adamczyk B, Węgrzyn K, Wilczyński T, et al. (2021) The most common lesions detected by neuroimaging as causes of epilepsy. *Medicina,* 57, 1–13.
136. Sharma S, Anand A, Garg D, et al. (2020) Use of the International League Against Epilepsy (ILAE) 1989, 2010, and 2017 classification of epilepsy in children in a low-resource setting: A hospital-based cross-sectional study. *Epilepsia Open,* 5, 397–405.
137. Syvertsen M, Nakken KO, Edland A, et al. (2015) Prevalence and etiology of epilepsy in a Norwegian county—A population based study. *Epilepsia,* 56, 699–706.
138. Wirrell E (2020) *Structural causes of epilepsy.* [online] Available at: <https://www.epilepsy.com/causes/structural> [Accessed September 20 2024].
139. Zuberi SM, Wirrell E, Yozawitz E, et al. (2022) ILAE classification and definition of epilepsy syndromes with onset in neonates and infants: Position statement by the ILAE Task Force on Nosology and Definitions. *Epilepsia,* 63, 1349–1397.
140. Rastin C, Schenkel LC, Sadikovic B (2023) Complexity in genetic epilepsies: A comprehensive review. *Int J Mol Sci,* 24, 1–17.
141. Wirrell E (2024) *Genetic causes of epilepsy.* [online] Available at: <https://www.epilepsy.com/causes/genetic> [Accessed September 20 2024].
142. Vezzani A, Fujinami RS, White HS, et al. (2016) Infections, inflammation and epilepsy. *Acta Neuropathol,* 131, 211–234.
143. Yacubian EMT, Kakooza-Mwesige A, Singh G, et al. (2022) Common infectious and parasitic diseases as a cause of seizures: Geographic distribution and contribution to the burden of epilepsy. *Epileptic Disord,* 24, 994–1019.
144. Preux PM, Druet-Cabanac M (2005) Epidemiology and aetiology of epilepsy in sub-Saharan Africa. *Lancet Neurol,* 4, 21–31.
145. Singhi P (2011) Infectious causes of seizures and epilepsy in the developing world. *Dev Med Child Neurol,* 53, 600–609.

146. Wilson MR, Sample HA, Zorn KC, et al. (2019) Clinical metagenomic sequencing for diagnosis of meningitis and encephalitis. *New England Journal of Medicine,* 380, 2327–2340.
147. Lin Lin Lee V, Kar Meng Choo B, Chung YS, et al. (2018) Treatment, therapy and management of metabolic epilepsy: A systematic review. *Int J Mol Sci,* 19, 1–20.
148. Almannai M, Al Mahmoud RA, Mekki M, El-Hattab AW (2021) Metabolic seizures. *Front Neurol,* 12, 1–14.
149. Sharma P, Hussain A, Greenwood R (2019) Precision in pediatric epilepsy. *F1000Res,* 8, 1–14.
150. Gavrilovici C, Rho JM (2021) Metabolic epilepsies amenable to ketogenic therapies: Indications, contraindications, and underlying mechanisms. *J Inherit Metab Dis,* 44, 42–53.
151. Husari KS, Dubey D (2019) Autoimmune epilepsy. *Neurotherapeutics,* 16, 685–702.
152. Chen TS, Lai MC, Huang HI, Wu SN, Huang CW (2022) Immunity, ion channels and epilepsy. *Int J Mol Sci,* 23.
153. Symonds JD, Elliott KS, Shetty J, et al. (2021) Early childhood epilepsies: Epidemiology, classification, aetiology, and socio-economic determinants. *Brain,* 144, 2879–2891.
154. Wirrell EC, Grossardt BR, Wong-Kisiel LC, Nickels KC (2011) Incidence and classification of new-onset epilepsy and epilepsy syndromes in children in Olmsted County, Minnesota from 1980 to 2004: A population-based study. *Epilepsy Res,* 95, 110–108.
155. Centers for Disease Control and Prevention (2024) *CDC's developmental milestones.* [online] Available at: <https://www.cdc.gov/ncbddd/actearly/milestones/index.html> [Accessed September 25 2024].
156. Wirrell E (2023) *Epilepsy syndromes—updated classifications and clinical management guidelines.* [online] Available at: <https://www.ilae.org/congresses/webinars/epilepsy-syndromes-updated-classifications-and-clinical-management-guidelines> [Accessed September 25 2024].
157. Raga S, Specchio N, Rheims S, Wilmshurst JM (2021) Developmental and epileptic encephalopathies: Recognition and approaches to care. *Epileptic Disord,* 23, 40–52.
158. International League Against Epilepsy (2024) *West syndrome.* [online] Available at: <https://epilepsydiagnosis.org/> [Accessed September 25 2024].
159. Hernandez A, Wirrell E (2020) *Infantile spasms West syndrome.* [online] Available at: <https://www.epilepsy.com/what-is-epilepsy/syndromes/infantile-spasms-west-syndrome> [Accessed September 25 2024].
160. Paprocka J, Malkiewicz J, Palazzo-Michalska V, et al. (2022) Effectiveness of ACTH in patients with infantile spasms. *Brain Sci,* 12, 1–15.
161. Nariai H, Duberstein S, Shinnar S (2018) Treatment of epileptic encephalopathies: Current state of the art. *J Child Neurol,* 33, 41–54.
162. International League Against Epilepsy (2024) *Dravet syndrome.* [online] Available at: <epilepsydiagnosis.org> [Accessed September 25 2024].

163. Epilepsy Foundation (2020) *Dravet syndrome*. [online] Available at: <https://www.epilepsy.com/what-is-epilepsy/syndromes/dravet-syndrome> [Accessed September 25 2024].
164. Wirrell EC, Hood V, Knupp KG, et al. (2022) International consensus on diagnosis and management of Dravet syndrome. *Epilepsia*, 63, 1761–1777.
165. Brodie MJ (2017) Sodium channel blockers in the treatment of epilepsy. *CNS Drugs*, 31, 527–534.
166. Sánchez-Espino LF, Ivars M, Antoñanzas J, Baselga E (2023) Sturge-Weber syndrome: A review of pathophysiology, genetics, clinical features, and current management approach. *Appl Clin Genet*, 16, 63–81.
167. International League Against Epilepsy (2024) *Sturge-Weber syndrome*. [online] Available at: <https://www.epilepsydiagnosis.org/aetiology/sturge-weber-genetics> [Accessed September 24 2024].
168. Specchio N, Wirrell EC, Scheffer IE, et al. (2022) International League Against Epilepsy classification and definition of epilepsy syndromes with onset in childhood: Position paper by the ILAE Task Force on Nosology and Definitions. *Epilepsia*, 63, 1398–1442.
169. International League Against Epilepsy (2024) *Epilepsy with myoclonic atonic seizures (EMAtS)*. [online] Available at: <https://www.epilepsydiagnosis.org/syndrome/epilepsy-myoclonic-atonic-genetics.html> [Accessed September 25 2024].
170. International League Against Epilepsy (2024) *Lennox Gastaut syndrome (LGS)*. [online] Available at: <https://www.epilepsydiagnosis.org/syndrome/lgs-overview.html> [Accessed September 25 2024].
171. Amrutkar CV, Riel-Romero RM (2023) *Lennox Gastaut Syndrome*. [e-book] Treasure Island (FL), StatPearls. Available at: National Library of Medicine <https://www.ncbi.nlm.nih.gov/books/NBK532965/> [Accessed September 25 2024].
172. Kiriakopoulos E, Wirrell E, Sirven JI, Osborne Shafer P (2024) *Lennox Gastaut syndrome LGS*. [online] Available at: <https://www.epilepsy.com/what-is-epilepsy/syndromes/lennox-gastaut-syndrome#What-is-Lennox-Gastaut-syndrome> [Accessed September 25 2024].
173. Epilepsy Foundation (2024) *LGS Foundation Lennox-Gastaut syndrome [pdf]*. [online] Available at: <https://www.epilepsy.com/sites/default/files/atoms/files/2019%20LGSF%20Fact%20Sheet%20FINAL%20%28 orignal%20version%29.pdf> [Accessed September 25 2024].
174. Muzio MR, Cascella M, Al Khalili Y (2023) *Landau-Kleffner Syndrome*. [e-book] Treasure Island (FL), StatPearls. Available at: National Library of Medicine <https://www.ncbi.nlm.nih.gov/books/NBK547745/> [Accessed September 25 2024].
175. National Organization for Rare Disorders (2023) *Landau Kleffner syndrome*. [online] Available at: <https://rarediseases.org/rare-diseases/landau-kleffner-syndrome/> [Accessed September 25 2024].
176. Clark M, Holmes H, Ngoh A, Siyani V, Wilson G (2021) Overview of Landau–Kleffner syndrome: Early treatment, tailored education and therapy improve outcome. *J Paediatr Child Health*, 31, 207–219.

177. Genetic and Rare Diseases Information Center (2024) *Landau-Kleffner syndrome*. [online] Available at: <https://rarediseases.info.nih.gov/diseases/6855/landau-kleffner-syndrome> [Accessed September 25 2024].
178. International League Against Epilepsy (2024) *Childhood absence epilepsy (CAE)*. [online] Available at: <https://www.epilepsydiagnosis.org/syndrome/cae-overview.html> [Accessed September 25 2024].
179. Kessler SK, Mcginnis E (2019) A practical guide to treatment of childhood absence epilepsy. *Paediatr Drugs*, 21, 15–24.
180. Holmes GL, Fisher R (2020) *Childhood absence epilepsy*. [online] Available at: <https://www.epilepsy.com/what-is-epilepsy/syndromes/childhood-absence-epilepsy> [Accessed September 25 2025].
181. Hirsch E, French J, Scheffer IE, et al. (2022) ILAE definition of the idiopathic generalized epilepsy syndromes: Position statement by the ILAE Task Force on Nosology and Definitions. *Epilepsia*, 63, 1475–1499.
182. Dagar A, Falcone T (2020) Psychiatric comorbidities in pediatric epilepsy. *Curr Psychiatry Rep*, 22, 1–10.
183. Boesen MS, Børresen ML, Christensen SK, et al. (2023) School performance and psychiatric comorbidity in childhood absence epilepsy: A Danish cohort study. *Eur J Paediatr Neurol*, 42, 75–81.
184. Vorderwülbecke BJ, Wandschneider B, Weber Y, Holtkamp M (2022) Genetic generalized epilepsies in adults—challenging assumptions and dogmas. *Nat Rev Neurol*, 18, 71–83.
185. International League Against Epilepsy (2024) *Juvenile absence epilepsy (JAE)*. [online] Available at: <https://www.epilepsydiagnosis.org/syndrome/jae-overview.html> [Accessed September 25 2024].
186. Yadala S, Nalleballe K (2023) *Juvenile Absence Epilepsy*. [e-book] Treasure Island (FL), StatPearls. Available at: National Library of Medicine <https://www.ncbi.nlm.nih.gov/books/NBK559055/> [Accessed September 24 2024].
187. International League Against Epilepsy (2024) *Juvenile myoclonic epilepsy (JME): Overview*. [online] Available at: <https://www.epilepsydiagnosis.org/syndrome/jme-overview.html> [Accessed September 25 2024].
188. Wirrell E (2019) *Juvenile Myoclonic Epilepsy*. [online] Available at: <https://www.epilepsy.com/what-is-epilepsy/syndromes/juvenile-myoclonic-epilepsy> [Accessed September 25 2024].
189. International League Against Epilepsy (2024) *Epilepsy with reading-induced seizures (EwRIS)*. [online] Available at: <https://www.epilepsydiagnosis.org/syndrome/reflex-epilepsies-overview.html> [Accessed September 25 2024].
190. Wylie T, Sandhu DS, Murr NI (2023) *Status Epilepticus*. [e-book] StatPearls. Available at: National Library of Medicine <https://www.ncbi.nlm.nih.gov/books/NBK430686/> [Accessed September 25 2024].
191. Mahler B, Carlsson S, Andersson T, Tomson T (2018) Risk for injuries and accidents in epilepsy: A prospective population-based cohort study. *Neurology*, 90, 779–789.
192. Strzelczyk A, Aledo-Serrano A, Coppola A, et al. (2023) The impact of epilepsy on quality of life: Findings from a European survey. *Epilepsy Behav*, 142, 1–11.

193. Hansebout RR, Cornacchi SD, Haines T, Goldsmith CH (2009) How to use an article about prognosis. *Can J Surg,* 52, 328–336.
194. Giussani G, Canelli V, Bianchi E, et al. (2016) Long-term prognosis of epilepsy, prognostic patterns and drug resistance: A population-based study. *Eur J Neurol,* 23, 1218–1227.
195. Centers for Disease Control and Prevention (2024) *About chronic diseases.* [online] Available at: <https://www.cdc.gov/chronic-disease/about/index.html> [Accessed September 25 2024].
196. Chen Z, Brodie MJ, Liew D, Kwan P (2018) Treatment outcomes in patients with newly diagnosed epilepsy treated with established and new antiepileptic drugs: A 30-year longitudinal cohort study. *JAMA Neurol,* 75, 279–286.
197. Sillanpää M, Schmidt D (2017) Long-term outcome of medically treated epilepsy. *Seizure,* 44, 211–216.
198. Löscher W, Klein P (2021) The pharmacology and clinical efficacy of antiseizure medications: From bromide salts to cenobamate and beyond. *CNS Drugs,* 35, 935–963.
199. Liu G, Slater N, Perkins A (2017) Epilepsy: Treatment options. *Am Fam Physician,* 96, 87–96.
200. Kwan P, Arzimanoglou A, Berg AT, et al. (2010) Definition of drug resistant epilepsy: Consensus proposal by the ad hoc Task Force of the ILAE Commission on Therapeutic Strategies. *Epilepsia,* 51, 1069-1077.
201. Wirrell E (2020) *Drug resistant epilepsy.* [online] Available at: <https://www.epilepsy.com/treatment/medicines/drug-resistant-epilepsy> [Accessed September 25 2024].
202. St Louis EK, Rosenfeld WE, Bramley T (2009) Antiepileptic drug monotherapy: The initial approach in epilepsy management. *Curr Neuropharmacol,* 7, 77–82.
203. Edinoff AN, Nix CA, Hollier J, et al. (2021) Benzodiazepines: Uses, dangers, and clinical considerations. *Neurol Int,* 13, 594–607.
204. Caffrey AR, Borrelli EP (2020) The art and science of drug titration. *Ther Adv Drug Saf,* 11, 1–14.
205. Obsorne Shafer P, Schachter SC (2022) *Seizure clusters.* [online] Available at: <https://www.epilepsy.com/complications-risks/emergencies/seizure-clusters> [Accessed September 25 2024].
206. Christian CA, Reddy DS, Maguire J, Forcelli PA (2020) Sex differences in the epilepsies and associated comorbidities: Implications for use and development of pharmacotherapies. *Pharmacol Rev,* 72, 767–800.
207. Wang J, Zhang J, Wu X, Yu P, Hong Z (2012) HLA-B*1502 allele is associated with a cross-reactivity pattern of cutaneous adverse reactions to antiepileptic drugs. *J Int Med Res,* 40, 377–382.
208. Sirven JI, Schachter SC (2013) *Side effects of seizure medicine.* [online] Available at: <https://www.epilepsy.com/treatment/medicines/side-effects> [Accessed September 25 2024].
209. Gabrielsson A, Tromans S, Watkins L, et al. (2023) Poo matters! A scoping review of the impact of constipation on epilepsy. *Seizure,* 108, 127–136.
210. Al-Beltagi M, Saeed NK (2022) Epilepsy and the gut: Perpetrator or victim? *World J Gastrointest Pathophysiol,* 13, 143–156.

211. Camfield P, Camfield C (2019) Regression in children with epilepsy. *Neurosci Biobehav Rev*, 96, 210–218.
212. Johnson E, Atkinson P, Muggeridge A, Cross JH, Reilly C (2022) Impact of epilepsy on learning and behaviour and needed supports: Views of children, parents and school staff. *Eur J Paediatr Neurol*, 40, 61–68.
213. Helmstaedter C, Sadat-Hossieny Z, Kanner AM, Meador KJ (2020) Cognitive disorders in epilepsy II: Clinical targets, indications and selection of test instruments. *Seizure*, 83, 223–231.
214. Chen B, Detyniecki K, Choi H, et al. (2017) Psychiatric and behavioral side effects of anti-epileptic drugs in adolescents and children with epilepsy. *Eur J Paediatr Neurol*, 21, 441–449.
215. Wei SH, Lee WT (2015) Comorbidity of childhood epilepsy. *J Formos Med Assoc*, 114, 1031–1038.
216. Abraham N, Buvanaswari P, Rathakrishnan R, et al. (2019) A meta-analysis of the rates of suicide ideation, attempts and deaths in people with epilepsy. *Int J Environ Res Public Health*, 16, 1–10.
217. Theochari EG, Cock HR (2019) Bone health in epilepsy. In: Mula M, ed., *The Comorbidities of Epilepsy*. London: Academic Press, pp 27–49.
218. Likasitthananon N, Nabangchang C, Simasathien T, et al. (2021) Hypovitaminosis D and risk factors in pediatric epilepsy children. *BMC Pediatr*, 21, 1–7.
219. Wang J, Huang P, Yu Q, et al. (2023) Epilepsy and long-term risk of arrhythmias. *Eur Heart J*, 44, 3374–3382.
220. American Heart Association (2023) *What is an arrhythmia [pdf]*. [online] Available at: <https://www.heart.org/-/media/files/health-topics/answers-by-heart/what-is-arrhythmia.pdf> [Accessed September 25 2024].
221. Ladino LD, Téllez-Zenteno JF (2019) Epilepsy and obesity: A complex interaction. In: Mula M, ed., *The Comorbidities of Epilepsy*. London: Academic Press, pp 131–158.
222. Sathyan A, Scaria R, Arunachalam P, et al. (2021) Antiepileptic drugs—induced enuresis in children: An overview. *J Pharm Technol*, 37, 114–119.
223. Oakley AM, Krishnamurthy K (2023) *Stevens-Johnson Syndrome*. [e-book] Treasure Island (FL), StatPearls. Available at: National Library of Medicine <https://www.ncbi.nlm.nih.gov/books/NBK459323/> [Accessed September 25 2024].
224. International League Against Epilepsy (2024) *Ketogenics diet basics*. [online] Available at: <https://www.ilae.org/patient-care/ketogenic-diets/basics> [Accessed September 25 2024].
225. Zhang Y, Xu J, Zhang K, Yang W, Li B (2018) The anticonvulsant effects of ketogenic diet on epileptic seizures and potential mechanisms. *Curr Neuropharmacol*, 16, 66–70.
226. Charlie Foundation for Ketogenic Therapies (2024) *Classic Keto*. [online] Available at: <https://charliefoundation.org/diet-plans/classic-keto/> [Accessed September 25 2024].

227. Sourbron J, Klinkenberg S, Van Kuijk SMJ, et al. (2020) Ketogenic diet for the treatment of pediatric epilepsy: Review and meta-analysis. *Childs Nerv Syst,* 36, 1099–1109.
228. Kossoff E (2007) *Side effects on the ketogenic diet: Identification and treatment.* [online] Available at: <https://www.epilepsy.com/stories/side-effects-ketogenic-diet-identification-and-treatment> [Accessed 2024 September 25].
229. Newmaster K, Zhu Z, Bolt E, et al. (2022) A review of the multi-systemic complications of a ketogenic diet in children and infants with epilepsy. *Children,* 9, 1–16.
230. Operto FF, Labate A, Aiello S, et al. (2023) The ketogenic diet in children with epilepsy: A focus on parental stress and family compliance. *Nutrients,* 15, 1–12.
231. Hidayatullah A (2019) The effectiveness of ketogenic diet in treatment of epilepsy patients: A literature review. *IJHNS,* 2, 39–44.
232. Hosain SA, La Vega-Talbott M, Solomon GE (2005) Ketogenic diet in pediatric epilepsy patients with gastrostomy feeding. *Pediatr Neurol,* 32, 81–83.
233. Ye F, Li XJ, Jiang WL, Sun HB, Liu J (2015) Efficacy of and patient compliance with a ketogenic diet in adults with intractable epilepsy: A meta-analysis. *J Clin Neurol,* 11, 26–31.
234. Neal EG, Chaffe H, Schwartz RH, et al. (2008) The ketogenic diet for the treatment of childhood epilepsy: A randomised controlled trial. *Lancet Neurol,* 7, 500–506.
235. Kossoff E (2017) *Ketogenic Diet.* [online] Available at: <https://www.epilepsy.com/treatment/dietary-therapies/ketogenic-diet#What-happens-first?> [Accessed September 25 2024].
236. Krames ES, Hunter Peckham P, Rezai A, Aboelsaad F (2009) What Is Neuromodulation? In: Krames ES, Hunter Peckham P, Rezai A, eds., *Neuromodulation.* San Diego: Academic Press, pp 3–8.
237. Kenny BJ, Bordoni B (2022) *Neuroanatomy, Cranial Nerve 10 (Valgus nerve).* [e-book] Treasure Island (FL), StatPearls. Available at: National Library of Medicine <https://www.ncbi.nlm.nih.gov/books/NBK537171/> [Accessed September 25 2024].
238. Shafer PO, Dean PM (2018) *Vagus nerve stimulation (VNS) therapy.* [online] Available at: <https://www.epilepsy.com/treatment/devices/vagus-nerve-stimulation-therapy> [Accessed September 25 2024].
239. González HFJ, Yengo-Kahn A, Englot DJ (2019) Vagus nerve stimulation for the treatment of epilepsy. *Neurosurg Clin N Am,* 30, 219–230.
240. Englot DJ, Hassnain KH, Rolston JD, et al. (2017) Quality-of-life metrics with vagus nerve stimulation for epilepsy from provider survey data. *Epilepsy Behav,* 66, 4–9.
241. Gillette Children's (2024) *Vagus nerve stimulation.* [online] Available at: <https://www.gillettechildrens.org/conditions-care/vagus-nerve-stimulation#what-to-expect-with-vagus-nerve-stimulation> [Accessed September 25 2024].
242. Mandalaneni K, Rayi A (eds.) 2023. *Vagus Nerve Stimulator,* Treasure Island (FL): StatPearls.
243. Shafer PO, Schachter SC (2018) *VNS therapy and travel.* [online] Available at: <https://www.epilepsy.com/lifestyle/travel/vns> [Accessed September 25 2024].

244. Iyengar S, Shafer PO (2017) *Responsive neurostimulation (RNS)*. [online] Available at: <https://www.epilepsy.com/treatment/devices/responsive-neurostimulation> [Accessed September 25 2024].
245. Singh RK, Eschbach K, Samanta D, et al. (2023) Responsive neurostimulation in drug-resistant pediatric epilepsy: Findings from the epilepsy surgery subgroup of the Pediatric Epilepsy Research Consortium. *Pediatr Neurol,* 143, 106–112.
246. Skarpaas TL, Jarosiewicz B, Morrell MJ (2019) Brain-responsive neurostimulation for epilepsy (RNS® System). *Epilepsy Res,* 153, 68–70.
247. Pierre L, Kondamudi NP (2023) *Subdural Hematoma.* [e-book] Treasure Island (FL), StatPearls. Available at: National Library of Medicine <https://www.ncbi.nlm.nih.gov/books/NBK532970/> [Accessed September 24 2024].
248. Razavi B, Rao VR, Lin C, et al. (2020) Real-world experience with direct brain-responsive neurostimulation for focal onset seizures. *Epilepsia,* 61, 1749–1757.
249. Kiriakopoulos E (2020) *Deep brain stimulation.* [online] Available at: <https://www.epilepsy.com/treatment/devices/deep-brain-stimulation> [Accessed September 25 2024].
250. Khan M, Paktiawal J, Piper RJ, Chari A, Tisdall MM (2022) Intracranial neuromodulation with deep brain stimulation and responsive neurostimulation in children with drug-resistant epilepsy: A systematic review. *J Neurosurg Pediatr,* 29, 208–217.
251. Li MCH, Cook MJ (2018) Deep brain stimulation for drug-resistant epilepsy. *Epilepsia,* 59, 273–290.
252. Salanova V, Witt T, Worth R, et al. (2015) Long-term efficacy and safety of thalamic stimulation for drug-resistant partial epilepsy. *Neurology,* 84, 1017–1025.
253. Crepeau AZ, Kiriakopoulos E (2023) *Risks and benefits of epilepsy surgery.* [online] Available at: <https://www.epilepsy.com/treatment/surgery/risks-and-benefits> [Accessed September 25 2024].
254. Baumgartner C, Koren JP, Britto-Arias M, Zoche L, Pirker S (2019) Presurgical epilepsy evaluation and epilepsy surgery. *F1000Res,* 8, 1–13.
255. Singh SP (2014) Magnetoencephalography: Basic principles. *Ann Indian Acad Neurol,* 17, 107–112.
256. Sirven JI, Kuzniecky R (2013) *MEG.* [online] Available at: <https://www.epilepsy.com/diagnosis/brain-imaging/magnetoencephalography> [Accessed September 25 2024].
257. Yandrapalli S, Puckett Y (2022) *SPECT Imaging.* [e-book] Treasure Island (FL), StatPearls. Available at: National Library of Medicine <https://www.ncbi.nlm.nih.gov/books/NBK564426/> [Accessed September 25 2024].
258. Sirven JI, Kuzniecky R (2013) *PET scan.* [online] Available at: <https://www.epilepsy.com/diagnosis/brain-imaging/pet> [Accessed September 25 2024].
259. Merriam-Webster (2024) *Uptake.* [online] Available at: <https://www.merriam-webster.com/dictionary/uptake> [Accessed September 25 2024].
260. Baxendale S, Wilson SJ, Baker GA, et al. (2019) Indications and expectations for neuropsychological assessment in epilepsy surgery in children and adults: Executive summary of the report of the ILAE Neuropsychology Task Force Diagnostic Methods Commission: 2017–2021. *Epilepsia,* 60, 1794–1796.

261. Al-Otaibi F, Baeesa SS, Parrent AG, Girvin JP, Steven D (2012) Surgical techniques for the treatment of temporal lobe epilepsy. *Epilepsy Res Treat*, 2012, 1–13.
262. Dallas J, Englot DJ, Naftel RP (2020) Neurosurgical approaches to pediatric epilepsy: Indications, techniques, and outcomes of common surgical procedures. *Seizure*, 77, 76–85.
263. Kiriakopoulos E, Cascino GD, Britton JW (2018) *Types of epilepsy surgery*. [online] Available at: <https://www.epilepsy.com/treatment/surgery/types#Temporal-Lobe-Resection> [Accessed September 25 2024].
264. Dwivedi R, Ramanujam B, Chandra PS, et al. (2017) Surgery for drug-resistant epilepsy in children. *NEJM*, 377, 1639–1647.
265. Maton B, Jayakar P, Resnick T, et al. (2008) Surgery for medically intractable temporal lobe epilepsy during early life. *Epilepsia*, 49, 80–87.
266. Wyllie E, Comair YG, Kotagal P, et al. (1998) Seizure outcome after epilepsy surgery in children and adolescents. *Ann Neurol*, 44, 740–748.
267. Hosoyama H, Matsuda K, Mihara T, et al. (2017) Long-term outcomes of epilepsy surgery in 85 pediatric patients followed up for over 10 years: A retrospective survey. *J Neurosurg Pediatr*, 19, 1–10.
268. Harris WB, Brunette-Clement T, Wang A, et al. (2022) Long-term outcomes of pediatric epilepsy surgery: Individual participant data and study level meta-analyses. *Seizure*, 101, 227–236.
269. Mehvari Habibabadi J, Moein H, Basiratnia R, et al. (2019) Outcome of lesional epilepsy surgery: Report of the first comprehensive epilepsy program in Iran. *Neurol Clin Pract*, 9, 286–295.
270. Lew SM (2014) Hemispherectomy in the treatment of seizures: A review. *Transl Pediatr*, 3, 208–217.
271. Kim JS, Park EK, Shim KW, Kim DS (2018) Hemispherotomy and functional hemispherectomy: Indications and outcomes. *J Epilepsy Res*, 8, 1–5.
272. Jaiswal V, Hanif M, Sarfraz Z, et al. (2021) Hemimegalencephaly: A rare congenital malformation of cortical development. *Clin Case Rep*, 9, 1–4.
273. Weil AG, Lewis EC, Ibrahim GM, et al. (2021) Hemispherectomy outcome prediction scale: Development and validation of a seizure freedom prediction tool. *Epilepsia*, 62, 1064–1073.
274. Gillette Children's (2024) *Corpus callostomy*. [online] Available at: <https://www.gillettechildrens.org/conditions-care/corpus-callosotomy> [Accessed September 25 2024].
275. Uda T, Kunihiro N, Umaba R, et al. (2021) Surgical aspects of corpus callosotomy. *Brain Sci*, 11, 3–8.
276. Graham D, Tisdall MM, Gill D (2016) Corpus callosotomy outcomes in pediatric patients: A systematic review. *Epilepsia*, 57, 1053–1068.
277. Asadi-Pooya AA, Sharan A, Nei M, Sperling MR (2008) Corpus callosotomy. *Epilepsy Behav*, 13, 271–278.
278. Dunoyer C, Ragheb J, Resnick T, et al. (2002) The use of stereotactic radiosurgery to treat intractable childhood partial epilepsy. *Epilepsia*, 43, 292–300.

279. Wei Z, Vodovotz L, Luy DD, et al. (2023) Stereotactic radiosurgery as the initial management option for small-volume hypothalamic hamartomas with intractable epilepsy: A 35-year institutional experience and systematic review. *J Neurosurg Pediatr,* 31, 52–60.
280. Ericson-Neilsen W, Kaye AD (2014) Steroids: Pharmacology, complications, and practice delivery issues. *Ochsner J,* 14, 203–207.
281. Zalkhani R, Moazedi A (2020) Basic and clinical role of vitamins in epilepsy. *J res appl basic med sci,* 6, 104–114.
282. Schachter SC (2024) *Nutritional deficiencies as a seizure trigger.* [online] Available at: <https://www.epilepsy.com/what-is-epilepsy/seizure-triggers/nutritional-deficiencies> [Accessed September 25 2024].
283. Romoli M, Perucca E, Sen A (2020) Pyridoxine supplementation for levetiracetam-related neuropsychiatric adverse events: A systematic review. *Epilepsy Behav,* 103, 1–5.
284. Yang MT, Chou IC, Wang HS (2023) Role of vitamins in epilepsy. *Epilepsy Behav,* 139, 1–6.
285. Das A, Sarwar MS, Hossain MS, et al. (2019) Elevated serum lipid peroxidation and reduced vitamin C and trace element concentrations are correlated with epilepsy. *Clin EEG Neurosci,* 50, 63–72.
286. Dong N, Guo HL, Hu YH, et al. (2022) Association between serum vitamin D status and the anti-seizure treatment in Chinese children with epilepsy. *Front Nutr,* 9, 1–17.
287. Upaganlawar AB, Wankhede NL, Kale MB, et al. (2021) Interweaving epilepsy and neurodegeneration: Vitamin E as a treatment approach. *Biomed Pharmacother,* 143, 1–12.
288. Zhu Z, Dluzynski D, Hammad N, et al. (2023) Use of integrative, complementary, and alternative medicine in children with epilepsy: A global scoping review. *Children,* 10, 1–23.
289. National Center for Complementary and Integrative Health (2019) *Cannabis (marijuana) and cannabinoids: What you need to know.* [online] Available at: <https://www.nccih.nih.gov/health/cannabis-marijuana-and-cannabinoids-what-you-need-to-know> [Accessed September 25 2024].
290. Lin CH, Hsieh CL (2021) Chinese herbal medicine for treating epilepsy. *Frontiers in Neuroscience,* 15, 1–13.
291. Devinsky O, Cross JH, Laux L, et al. (2017) Trial of cannabidiol for drug-resistant seizures in the Dravet syndrome. *N Engl J Med,* 376, 2011–2020.
292. Devinsky O, Patel AD, Cross JH, et al. (2018) Effect of cannabidiol on drop seizures in the Lennox-Gastaut syndrome. *N Engl J Med,* 378, 1888–1897.
293. Thiele EA, Bebin EM, Bhathal H, et al. (2021) Add-on cannabidiol treatment for drug-resistant seizures in tuberous sclerosis complex: A placebo-controlled randomized clinical trial. *JAMA Neurol,* 78, 285–292.
294. Sands TT, Rahdari S, Oldham MS, et al. (2019) Long-term safety, tolerability, and efficacy of cannabidiol in children with refractory epilepsy: Results from an expanded access program in the US. *CNS Drugs,* 33, 47–60.

295. National Center for Complementary and Integrative Health (2023) *Complementary, Alternative, or Integrative Health: What's In a Name?* [online] Available at: <https://www.nccih.nih.gov/health/complementary-alternative-or-integrative-health-whats-in-a-name> [Accessed April 23 2024].
296. Britannica Money (2024) *Developing country.* [online] Available at: <https://www.britannica.com/money/developing-country> [Accessed September 25 2024].
297. Zhao C, Lu L, Liu W, Zhou D, Wu X (2022) Complementary and alternative medicine for treating epilepsy in China: A systematic review. *Acta Neurol Scand*, 146, 775–785.
298. Nei M, Ngo L, Sirven JI, Sperling MR (2014) Ketogenic diet in adolescents and adults with epilepsy. *Seizure*, 23, 439–442.
299. Rezaei S, Harsini S, Kavoosi M, Badv RS, Mahmoudi M (2018) Efficacy of low glycemic index treatment in epileptic patients: A systematic review. *Acta Neurol Belg*, 118, 339–349.
300. Ahmadi F, Khalatbary AR (2021) A review on the neuroprotective effects of hyperbaric oxygen therapy. *Med Gas Res*, 11, 72–82.
301. Banham ND (2011) Oxygen toxicity seizures: 20 years' experience from a single hyperbaric unit. *Diving Hyperb Med*, 41, 202–210.
302. Manning EP (2016) Central nervous system oxygen toxicity and hyperbaric oxygen seizures. *Aerosp Med Hum Perform*, 87, 477–86.
303. Olschewski DN, Bauer PR, Sander JW (2019) The comorbidities of epilepsy: A conceptual framework. In: Mula M, ed., *The Comorbidities of Epilepsy*. London: Academic Press, pp 1–11.
304. Giussani G, Bianchi E, Beretta S, et al. (2021) Comorbidities in patients with epilepsy: Frequency, mechanisms and effects on long-term outcome. *Epilepsia*, 62, 2395–2404.
305. Morris-Rosendahl DJ, Crocq MA (2020) Neurodevelopmental disorders—the history and future of a diagnostic concept. *Dialogues Clin Neurosci*, 22, 65–72.
306. Rosenbaum P, Paneth N, Leviton A, et al. (2007) A report: the definition and classification of cerebral palsy April 2006. *Dev Med Child Neurol Suppl*, 109, 8–14.
307. Smithers-Sheedy H, Waight E, Goldsmith S, McIntyre S (2023) Australian Cerebral Palsy Register Report, Available at: <https://cpregister.com/wp-content/uploads/2023/01/2023-ACPR-Report.pdf> [Accessed June 24 2024].
308. Graham HK, Rosenbaum P, Paneth N, et al. (2016) Cerebral palsy. *Nat Rev Dis Primers*, 2, 1–24.
309. Pavone P, Gulizia C, Le Pira A, et al. (2020) Cerebral palsy and epilepsy in children: Clinical perspectives on a common comorbidity. *Children*, 8, 1–11.
310. Sadowska M, Sarecka-Hujar B, Kopyta I (2020) Evaluation of risk factors for epilepsy in pediatric patients with cerebral palsy. *Brain Sci*, 10.
311. American Psychiatric Association (2024) *What is intellectual disability?* [online] Available at: <https://www.psychiatry.org/patients-families/intellectual-disability> [Accessed July 27 2024].
312. Dhakal A, Bobrin BD (2023) *Cognitive Deficits*. [e-book] Treasure Island (FL), StatPearls Publishing. Available at: National Library of Medicine <https://www.ncbi.nlm.nih.gov/books/NBK559052/> [Accessed September 25 2024].

313. National Institute of Neurological Disorders and Stroke (2024) *Learning disabilities*. [online] Available at: <https://www.ninds.nih.gov/health-information/disorders/learning-disabilities> [Accessed September 25 2024].
314. Brandt C (2019) Epilepsy and intellectual disabilities. In: Mula M, ed., *The Comorbidities of Epilepsy*. London: Academic Press, pp 273–284.
315. Semrud-Clikeman M, Teeter Ellison PA (2009) Introduction to child clinical neuropsychology. In: Semrud-Clikeman M, Teeter Ellison PA, eds., *Child Neuropsychology*. New York: Springer, pp 3–25.
316. National Institute of Mental Health (2024) *Attention-deficit/hyperactivity disorder*. [online] Available at: <https://www.nimh.nih.gov/health/topics/attention-deficit-hyperactivity-disorder-adhd> [Accessed September 25 2024].
317. Fan HC, Chiang KL, Chang KH, Chen CM, Tsai JD (2023) Epilepsy and attention deficit hyperactivity disorder: Connection, chance, and challenges. *Int J Mol Sci*, 24, 1–30.
318. Besag F, Aldenkamp A, Caplan R, et al. (2016) Psychiatric and behavioural disorders in children with epilepsy: An ILAE task force report. *Epileptic Disord*, 18, 1–86.
319. Chou IC, Chang YT, Chin ZN, et al. (2013) Correlation between epilepsy and attention deficit hyperactivity disorder: A population-based cohort study. *PLoS One*, 8, 1–5.
320. Ahmed GK, Darwish AM, Khalifa H, Haridy NA (2022) Relationship between attention deficit hyperactivity disorder and epilepsy: A literature review. *Egypt. J. Neurol. Psychiatry Neurosurg*, 58, 52.
321. Rheims S, Auvin S (2021) Attention deficit/hyperactivity disorder and epilepsy. *Curr Opin Neurol*, 34, 219–225.
322. Kanner AM, Helmstaedter C, Sadat-Hossieny Z, Meador K (2020) Cognitive disorders in epilepsy I: Clinical experience, real-world evidence and recommendations. *Seizure*, 83, 216–222.
323. Auvin S, Wirrell E, Donald KA, et al. (2018) Systematic review of the screening, diagnosis, and management of ADHD in children with epilepsy. Consensus paper of the Task Force on Comorbidities of the ILAE Pediatric Commission. *Epilepsia*, 59, 1867–1880.
324. Pavlova MK, Ng M, Allen RM, et al. (2021) Proceedings of the Sleep and Epilepsy Workgroup: Section 2 Comorbidities: Sleep Related Comorbidities of Epilepsy. *Epilepsy Curr*, 21, 210–214.
325. Giorelli AS, Passos P, Carnaval T, Gomes Mda M (2013) Excessive daytime sleepiness and epilepsy: A systematic review. *Epilepsy Res Treat*, 1–9.
326. Auvin S, Dozières-Puyravel B, Loussouarn A (2019) Epilepsy and autistic spectrum disorder: Diagnostic challenges and treatment consideration. In: Mula M, ed., *The Comorbidities of Epilepsy*. London: Academic Press, pp 285–297.
327. Liu X, Sun X, Sun C, et al. (2022) Prevalence of epilepsy in autism spectrum disorders: A systematic review and meta-analysis. *Autism*, 26, 33–50.
328. International Rett Syndrome Foundation (2024) *Frequently asked questions*. [online] Available at: <https://www.rettsyndrome.org/about-rett-syndrome/faqs/> [Accessed September 25 2024].

329. Saby JN, Peters SU, Roberts TPL, Nelson CA, Marsh ED (2020) Evoked potentials and EEG analysis in Rett syndrome and related developmental encephalopathies: Towards a biomarker for translational research. *Front Integr Neurosci*, 14, 1–12.
330. Genetic and Rare Diseases Information Center (2024) *Rett syndrome*. [online] Available at: <https://rarediseases.info.nih.gov/diseases/5696/rett-syndrome> [Accessed September 25 2024].
331. Operto FF, Mazza R, Pastorino GMG, Verrotti A, Coppola G (2019) Epilepsy and genetic in Rett syndrome: A review. *Brain Behav*, 9, 1–10.
332. Akhtar F, Rizwan S, Bokhari A (2023) *Down Syndrome*. [e-book] Treasure Island (FL), StatPearls. Available at: National Library of Medicine <https://www.ncbi.nlm.nih.gov/books/NBK526016/> [Accessed September 25 2024].
333. Altuna M, Giménez S, Fortea J (2021) Epilepsy in Down syndrome: A highly prevalent comorbidity. *J Clin Med*, 10, 1–17.
334. Rout P, Zamora EA, Aeddula NR (2024) *Tuberous Sclerosis*. [e-book] Treasure Island (FL), StatPearls. Available at: National Library of Medicine <https://www.ncbi.nlm.nih.gov/books/NBK538492/> [Accessed September 25, 2024].
335. Schubert-Bast S, Strzelczyk A (2021) Review of the treatment options for epilepsy in tuberous sclerosis complex: Towards precision medicine. *Ther Adv Neurol Disord*, 14, 1–22.
336. Aaberg KM, Bakken IJ, Lossius MI, et al. (2016) Comorbidity and childhood epilepsy: A nationwide registry study. *Pediatrics*, 138, 1–10.
337. Keezer MR, Sisodiya SM, Sander JW (2016) Comorbidities of epilepsy: Current concepts and future perspectives. *Lancet Neurol*, 15, 106–115.
338. Durá-Travé T, Gallinas-Victoriano F, Malumbres-Chacón M, et al. (2018) Vitamin D deficiency in children with epilepsy taking valproate and levetiracetam as monotherapy. *Epilepsy Res*, 139, 80–84.
339. Diemar SS, Sejling AS, Eiken P, Andersen NB, Jørgensen NR (2019) An explorative literature review of the multifactorial causes of osteoporosis in epilepsy. *Epilepsy Behav*, 100, 1–10.
340. Arora E, Singh H, Gupta YK (2016) Impact of antiepileptic drugs on bone health: Need for monitoring, treatment, and prevention strategies. *J Family Med Prim Care*, 5, 248–253.
341. Subbararo BS, Silverman A, Eapen BC (2023) *Seizure Medications*. [e-book] Treasure Island (FL), StatPearls. Available at: National Library of Medicine <https://www.ncbi.nlm.nih.gov/books/NBK482269/> [Accessed September 25 2024].
342. Costagliola G, Orsini A, Coll M, et al. (2021) The brain-heart interaction in epilepsy: Implications for diagnosis, therapy, and SUDEP prevention. *Ann Clin Transl Neurol*, 8, 1557–1568.
343. Eggleston KS, Olin BD, Fisher RS (2014) Ictal tachycardia: The head-heart connection. *Seizure*, 23, 496–505.
344. Wright EC, Mitchell L, Hewett R, Anderton L (2021) Ictal asystole: An uncommon but significant cause of transient loss of consciousness—a case series. *BMJ Case Rep*, 14, 1–4.
345. Kim JB (2014) Channelopathies. *Korean J Pediatr*, 57, 1–18.

346. Al-Akchar M, Siddique MS (2024) *Long QT Syndrome*. [e-book] Treasure Island (FL), StatPearls. Available at: National Library of Medicine <https://pubmed.ncbi.nlm.nih.gov/28722890/>.
347. Marstrand P, Theilade J, Andersson C, et al. (2019) Long QT syndrome is associated with an increased burden of diabetes, psychiatric and neurological comorbidities: A nationwide cohort study. *Open Heart*, 6, 1–8.
348. Harvey S, King MD, Gorman KM (2021) Paroxysmal movement disorders. *Front Neurol*, 12, 1–16.
349. De Gusmão CM, Garcia L, Mikati MA, Su S, Silveira-Moriyama L (2021) Paroxysmal genetic movement disorders and epilepsy. *Front Neurol*, 12, 1–16.
350. Avorio F, Cerulli Irelli E, Morano A, et al. (2021) Functional gastrointestinal disorders in patients with epilepsy: Reciprocal influence and impact on seizure occurrence. *Frontiers in Neurology*, 12.
351. Amanat M, Thijs RD, Salehi M, Sander JW (2019) Seizures as a clinical manifestation in somatic autoimmune disorders. *Seizure*, 64, 59–64.
352. World Health Organization (2023) *Depressive disorder (depression)*. [online] Available at: <https://www.who.int/news-room/fact-sheets/detail/depression> [Accessed September 25 2024].
353. World Health Organization (2023) *Anxiety disorders*. [online] Available at: <https://www.who.int/news-room/fact-sheets/detail/anxiety-disorders> [Accessed September 25 2024].
354. Scott AJ, Sharpe L, Loomes M, Gandy M (2020) Systematic review and meta-analysis of anxiety and depression in youth with epilepsy. *J Pediatr Psychol*, 45, 133–144.
355. Centers for Disease Control and Prevention (2023) *Data and statistics on children's mental health*. [online] Available at: <https://www.cdc.gov/childrensmentalhealth/data.html> [Accessed September 25 2024].
356. Mora Rodríguez K, Benbadis S (2016) *Epilepsy and psychological disorders*. [online] Available at: <https://www.epilepsy.com/stories/epilepsy-and-psychological-disorders> [Accessed September 25 2024].
357. Dunn DW, Besag F, Caplan R, et al. (2016) Psychiatric and behavioural disorders in children with epilepsy (ILAE Task Force Report): Anxiety, depression and childhood epilepsy. *Epileptic Disord*, 18, 24–30.
358. Kanner AM (2022) Suicidality in patients with epilepsy: Why should neurologists care? *Front Integr Neurosci*, 16, 1–8.
359. Leppien EE, Doughty BJ, Hurd KL, et al. (2023) Newer antiseizure medications and suicidality: Analysis of the Food and Drug Administration Adverse Event Reporting System (FAERS) Database. *Clin Drug Investig*, 43, 393–399.
360. Aggarwal A, Marwaha R (2022) *Oppositional Defiant Disorder*. [e-book] Treasure Island (FL), StatPearls. Available at: National Library of Medicine <https://www.ncbi.nlm.nih.gov/books/NBK557443/>.
361. Brock H, Rizvi I, Hany M (2024) *Obsessive-Compulsive Disorder*. [e-book] Treasure Island (FL), StatPearls. Available at: National Library of Medicine <https://www.ncbi.nlm.nih.gov/books/NBK553162/> [Accessed September 25 2024].

362. Epilepsy Foundation (2022) *Epilepsy and OCD*. [online] Available at: <https://www.epilepsy.com/complications-risks/moods-behavior/ocd> [Accessed September 25 2024].
363. Mohan L, Yilani M, Ray S (2023) *Conduct disorder*. [online] Available at: <https://www.ncbi.nlm.nih.gov/books/NBK470238/> [Accessed September 25 2024].
364. Sillanpää M, Besag F, Aldenkamp A, et al. (2016) Psychiatric and behavioural disorders in children with epilepsy (ILAE Task Force Report): Epidemiology of psychiatric/behavioural disorder in children with epilepsy. *Epileptic Disord*, 18, 2–7.
365. Whitson J, Agrawal N (2019) Epilepsy and psychosis. In: Mula M, ed., *The Comorbidities of Epilepsy*. London: Academic Press, pp 315–342.
366. Peters J, Vijiaratnam N, Angus-Leppan H (2021) Tics induced by antiepileptic drugs: A pragmatic review. *J Neurol*, 268, 321–336.
367. Abdullahi A, Taura U, Farouk Z (2019) The role of school in the management of children with epilepsy. *J Health Res Rev Dev*, 6, 37–41.
368. Guilfoyle SM, Wagner JL, Modi AC, et al. (2017) Pediatric epilepsy and behavioral health: The state of the literature and directions for evidence-based interprofessional care, training, and research. *Clinical Practice in Pediatric Psychology*, 5, 79–90.
369. Modi AC, Ingerski LM, Rausch JR, Glauser TA (2011) Treatment factors affecting longitudinal quality of life in new onset pediatric epilepsy. *J Pediatr Psychol*, 36, 466–475.
370. Eze CN, Ebuehi OM, Brigo F, Otte WM, Igwe SC (2015) Effect of health education on trainee teachers' knowledge, attitudes, and first aid management of epilepsy: An interventional study. *Seizure*, 33, 46–53.
371. Prasad V, Kendrick D, Sayal K, Thomas SL, West J (2014) Injury among children and young adults with epilepsy. *Pediatrics*, 133, 827–835.
372. Lagunju IA, Oyinlade AO, Babatunde OD (2016) Seizure-related injuries in children and adolescents with epilepsy. *Epilepsy Behav*, 54, 131–134.
373. Ripatti L, Puustinen L, Rautava P, Koivisto M, Haataja L (2023) Impact of epilepsy on the risk of hospital-treated injuries in Finnish children. *Epilepsy Behav Rep*, 21, 1–5.
374. Cuello Oderiz C (2015) *Epilepsy and driving*. [online] Available at: <https://www.epilepsy.com/stories/epilepsy-and-driving> [Accessed September 25 2024].
375. McLachlan RS, Starreveld E, Lee MA (2007) Impact of mandatory physician reporting on accident risk in epilepsy. *Epilepsia*, 48, 1500–1505.
376. Kaur J, Paul BS, Goel P, Singh G (2019) Educational achievement, employment, marriage, and driving in adults with childhood-onset epilepsy. *Epilepsy Behav*, 97, 149–153.
377. Koppel S, Di Stefano M, Dimech-Betancourt B, et al. (2021) What is the motor vehicle crash risk for drivers with epilepsy? A systematic review. *Journal of Transport & Health*, 23, 1–20.
378. Capovilla G, Kaufman KR, Perucca E, Moshé SL, Arida RM (2016) Epilepsy, seizures, physical exercise, and sports: A report from the ILAE Task Force on Sports and Epilepsy. *Epilepsia*, 57, 6–12.

379. Pimentel J, Tojal R, Morgado J (2015) Epilepsy and physical exercise. *Seizure,* 25, 87–94.
380. Sirven JI, Osborne Shafer P, Fisher R (2013) *Staying safe.* [online] Available at: <https://www.epilepsy.com/preparedness-safety/staying-safe> [Accessed September 25 2024].
381. Burckhardt CS, Anderson KL (2003) The Quality of Life Scale (QOLS): Reliability, validity, and utilization. *Health Qual Life Outcomes,* 1, 1–7.
382. U.S. Department of Education (2024) *Individuals with Disabilities Education Act.* [online] Available at: <https://sites.ed.gov/idea/> [Accessed September 25 2024].
383. Puka K, Tavares TP, Speechley KN (2019) Social outcomes for adults with a history of childhood-onset epilepsy: A systematic review and meta-analysis. *Epilepsy Behav,* 92, 297–305.
384. Epilepsy Foundation (2024) *Pilots and epilepsy.* [online] Available at: <https://www.epilepsy.com/lifestyle/employment/pilot> [Accessed September 25 2024].
385. Smart D, Lippmann J (2013) Epilepsy, scuba diving and risk assessment. Near misses and the need for ongoing vigilance. *Diving Hyperb Med,* 43, 37–41.
386. Division USDOJCR (2024) *Introduction to the Americans with Disabilities Act.* [online] Available at: <https://www.ada.gov/topics/intro-to-ada/> [Accessed September 25 2024].
387. Got Transition (2024) *Six core elements of health care transition.* [online] Available at: <https://www.gottransition.org/six-core-elements/> [Accessed September 25 2024].
388. Meyers MJ, Irwin CE (2023) Health care transitions for adolescents. *Pediatrics,* 151, 1–5.
389. Schmidt A, Ilango SM, McManus MA, Rogers KK, White PH (2020) Outcomes of pediatric to adult health care transition interventions: An updated systematic review. *J Pediatr Nurs,* 51, 92–107.
390. Kirkpatrick L, Collins A, Sogawa Y, et al. (2020) Sexual and reproductive healthcare for adolescent and young adult women with epilepsy: A qualitative study of pediatric neurologists and epileptologists. *Epilepsy Behav,* 104, 1–6.
391. World Health Organization (2024) *Contraception.* [online] Available at: <https://www.who.int/health-topics/contraception> [Accessed September 25 2024].
392. Manski R, Dennis A (2014) A mixed-methods exploration of the contraceptive experiences of female teens with epilepsy. *Seizure,* 23, 629–35.
393. Gaffield ME, Culwell KR, Lee CR (2011) The use of hormonal contraception among women taking anticonvulsant therapy. *Contraception,* 83, 16–29.
394. Atif M, Sarwar MR, Scahill S (2016) The relationship between epilepsy and sexual dysfunction: A review of the literature. *Springerplus,* 5, 1–10.
395. Mann C, Süß A, Von Podewils F, et al. (2022) Gender differences in concerns about planning to have children and child-rearing among patients with epilepsy: A prospective, multicenter study with 477 patients from Germany. *Epilepsy Behav,* 129, 1–5.
396. Sureja P (2014) *Epilepsy and pregnancy: Frequently asked questions.* [online] Available at: <https://www.epilepsy.com/stories/epilepsy-and-pregnancy-frequently-asked-questions> [Accessed September 25 2024].

397. Reimers A, Brodtkorb E, Sabers A (2015) Interactions between hormonal contraception and antiepileptic drugs: Clinical and mechanistic considerations. *Seizure*, 28, 66–70.
398. Herzog AG, Mandle HB, Cahill KE, Fowler KM, Hauser WA (2017) Predictors of unintended pregnancy in women with epilepsy. *Neurology*, 88, 728–733.
399. Adamolekun B (2024) *Antiseizure medications*. [online] Available at: <https://www.merckmanuals.com/professional/neurologic-disorders/seizure-disorders/antiseizure-medications?ruleredirectid=747> [Accessed September 25 2024].
400. Nucera B, Brigo F, Trinka E, Kalss G (2022) Treatment and care of women with epilepsy before, during, and after pregnancy: A practical guide. *Ther Adv Neurol Disord*, 15, 1–31.
401. Patel SI, Pennell PB (2016) Management of epilepsy during pregnancy: An update. *Ther Adv Neurol Disord*, 9, 118–129.
402. Li Y, Meador KJ (2022) Epilepsy and pregnancy. *Continuum*, 28, 34–54.
403. Simon LV, Hashmi MF, Bragg BN (2023) *APGAR Score*. [e-book] Treasure Island (FL), StatPearls Publishing. Available at: National Library of Medicine <https://www.ncbi.nlm.nih.gov/books/NBK542197/> [Accessed March 29 2024].
404. Herzog AG, Mandle HB, MacEachern DB (2019) Association of unintended pregnancy with spontaneous fetal loss in women with epilepsy: Findings of the Epilepsy Birth Control Registry. *JAMA Neurol*, 76, 50–55.
405. World Health Organization (2024) *Infertility*. [online] Available at: <https://www.who.int/news-room/fact-sheets/detail/infertility> [Accessed September 25 2024].
406. MacEachern DB, Mandle HB, Herzog AG (2019) Infertility, impaired fecundity, and live birth/pregnancy ratio in women with epilepsy in the USA: Findings of the Epilepsy Birth Control Registry. *Epilepsia*, 60, 1993–1998.
407. Lackey AE, Muzio MR (2023) *DiGeorge Syndrome*. [e-book] Treasure Island (FL), StatPearls. Available at: National Library of Medicine <https://www.ncbi.nlm.nih.gov/books/NBK549798/> [Accessed September 25 2024].

Index

Figures and tables indicated by page numbers in italics.

A
absence seizures, 36, 37–38, *38*
ACTH (adrenocorticotropic hormone therapy), *51,* 200
activities, restricted by epilepsy, 236, 238–244
ADHD (attention deficit hyperactivity disorder), 219–220
alternative therapies, 205–208
amygdala, 68, *69*
antiseizure medications
  about, 168–181, *172, 177*
  adverse side effects, 168, 171, 179–180, 206, 213, 225, 231, 253–254, 255
  ongoing *versus* seizure rescue, 171–173
  and pregnancy, 253–255
  remission and resolution, 167, 170
  and seizure threshold, 73
  and vitamins, 201
anxiety, 229–230, 231, 236
aphasia, 67
Atkins diet, modified, 207
atonic events, 34, 36–37
auras, 18–19, 35
autism spectrum disorder, 10, 221
autoimmune dysregulation conditions, 110
automatisms, 34
autonomic actions, 35
autonomic nervous system disorders, 227
awareness, during seizure, 32–33

B
behavioral arrest, 35
behavioral disorders, 229–231
benign convulsions, and gastroenteritis, 9
bipolar disorder, 231
bipolar montage, 84, *85*

birth control, hormonal, 178, 253–254
blood cell count, 109
brain. *See also* nervous system
  about, 61–69, *62, 63, 64, 67, 68, 69*
  cerebrovascular conditions, 19, 107
  damage from epilepsy, 165, 166
  imaging, 106–107
  and seizure onset zone, 31–32
  and seizures, 4
brain stem, 62, *62*
breakthrough seizures, 165, 173, 176, 177, *177*
Broca's area, 67, *68*

C
cannabis, medical, *51,* 201–202
cardiovascular system disorders, 19, 107, 225–226
career planning, 245, 246–247
case studies, 292–293
central nervous system, *59, 60*
cerebellum, 62, *62*
cerebral cortex, 61–62, *63,* 63–67, *64*
cerebral palsy, and epilepsy, 10, 217
cerebrospinal fluid, 110, 112
cerebrovascular conditions, 19, 107
cerebrum, 61–62, *62*
channelopathies, 226
childhood absence epilepsy (CAE), 153
clinical seizures, 89
clinical trials, 293–294
clonic movements, 34, 37
cognitive impairment, 219
cognitive symptoms, 35
cohort study, 292
combined generalized and focal epilepsy, 45

comorbidities
    about, 46, 213–215, *215*
    and antiseizure medication, 178, 179–180
    neurological and neurodevelopmental, 216–221
    physical, 224–227
    psychiatric, 229–231
    psychosocial impact, 237
complementary therapies, 205–208
conduct disorder (CD), 231
contraceptives, oral, 178, 253–254
convulsions (benign), and gastroenteritis, 9
corpus callosum, 62, *63,* 196–197
cross-sectional study, 292
CT (computed tomography), 106–107, 194

D

decision-making, shared, 52
deep brain stimulation, *192,* 192–193
depression, 229–230, 231
developmental and epileptic encephalopathies (DEEs), 143–145, 150
developmental delay, 141, 143, 150, 218
discrimination, 246
dogs, and seizure detection, 98–99
Down syndrome, 221
Dravet syndrome, 144–145
driver's license, 239–240, 246
drop seizures, 34, 37
drug-resistant epilepsy, 169–170. See also non-pharmaceutical treatments

E

ECG (electrocardiogram), *81,* 85
education, for people with epilepsy, 245–246
EEG (electroencephalography)
    about, 79
    description of test process, 80–85, *81, 83, 84, 85*
    as diagnostic test, 79, 89–90, 122
    interpretation, 86–90, *91*
    phases of a seizure, 92–93, *94*
    before surgery, 193–194
electrographic seizures, 89–90
electrolyte levels, 109
EMG (electromyography), 85
emotional symptoms, 35
employment, rates of, 246
encephalitis, 127
epilepsy. *See also* antiseizure medications; comorbidities; *seizure entries*
    about, 3–11

and age, 10, 11, 49
causes and risk factors, 9–10, 45, 106, 121–133, *122*
classification, 43–46, *44, 122*
definition, 4–5
diagnosis, 15, 27, 29–30, 89–90, 105–116 (*see also* EEG [electroencephalography]; epilepsy syndromes)
and genetics, 45, 115–116, 125–126
prevalence, 10–11, 124, 125, 127–128, 129, 133
prognosis, 166–167
psychosocial impact, 236–237
epilepsy, management
    about, 48–52, *51,* 163–164
    alternative/complementary therapies, 205–208
    and comorbidities, 215
    detecting and recording seizures, 95–99
    determined by syndrome, 139
    diet, 183–187, 207
    goals of, 164–166
    non-pharmaceutical treatments, 182–198
    and other illnesses, 180–181
    other medications, 199–200
    pharmaceutical, 168–181, *172, 177*
    and pregnancy, 254–255
    risk of injury, 238–239, *241*
    supplements, 200–202, 206–207
    transition from childhood to adulthood, 52, 249–250, *251, 252*
epilepsy syndromes
    about, 4–5, 45–46, 139–141
    in adolescence and adulthood, 154–156
    in childhood, 149–153
    in neonatal period and infancy, 142–146
    onset at variable age, 157–158
epileptic spasms, 34, 37
epileptiform discharges, 88, 89–90
etiology-specific epilepsy syndromes, 145–146
evidence-based medicine, 52, 250, 289–290
exercise, 240
extratemporal cortical resection, 195–196

F

families, engagement in research, 293–295
family-centered care, 52, 249
family planning, 253–255
febrile seizures, 8–9, 10, 16

females
   and antiseizure medication, 178, 253–254
   and birth control, 178, 253–254
   and epilepsy, 178, 221, 253
   and pregnancy, 254–255
first aid, for seizures, 12–14, *13*
focal epilepsy, 44
focal epilepsy syndromes, 154–155
focal onset seizures, 32, 34–36, *36, 40*
folic acid, 255
frontal lobe, 63, *64, 65,* 67. *See also* motor cortex

G
gastroenteritis, and benign convulsions, 9
gastroesophageal reflux disease (GERD), 16–17
generalized epilepsy, 45
generalized epilepsy syndromes, 152, 155–156
generalized onset seizures, 32, 36–38, *38, 40*
genetic epilepsy, 45, 125–126
genetic generalized epilepsy (GGE), 153, 155
genetic testing, 114–116, *115*

H
heart arrythmias, 85, 225–226
heart disease, 225
hemispherectomy, 196
herbal supplements, 206, 207
hippocampal sclerosis, 68, 123
hippocampus, 68, *69*
hyperbaric oxygen therapy, 207–208
hyperkinetic movements, 34
hypoglycemia, 17
hypsarrhythmia, 93

I
ictal epileptiform discharges, 88
ictal phase of seizure, 42, *42,* 92
immune dysregulation conditions, 110
immune epilepsy, 45, 131–132
immunotherapies, 51, 199
independence, 50, 99, 166, 218, 236, 249–250, *251*
infantile epileptic spasms syndrome (West syndrome), 144
infectious epilepsy, 45, 127–128
injuries, risk of, 238–239, *241*

intellectual disability, 218–219
interictal epileptiform discharges, 88, 90
interictal phase of seizure, 93
ion channels, 71, 178–179, 226

J
juvenile absence epilepsy (JAE), 153, 155
juvenile myoclonic epilepsy (JME), 153, 155–156

K
ketogenic diet, 51, 183–187, *184,* 201

L
laboratory tests, for diagnosis, 108–110
Landau-Kleffner syndrome, 152
learning disorders, 219
Lennox-Gestaut syndrome, 151–152
lesionectomy, 196
long QT syndrome, 226
low glycemic index treatment, 207
lumbar puncture, 112, *113*

M
males, and antiseizure medications, 254
meningitis, 127
metabolic epilepsy, 45, 129–130
metabolism evaluation, 110
migraines, 18, 220
mineral supplements, 206
monotherapy, 51, 169–170
motor cortex, 66, 67
motor signs, 33–34, *36,* 36–37, *38,* 66, 85
MRI (magnetic resonance imaging), 107, 194
multidisciplinary team approach, 52
musculoskeletal system disorders, 224–225
myoclonic-atonic movements, 37
myoclonic-atonic seizures, 151
myoclonic movements, 34, 37
myoclonic-tonic-clonic movements, 37

N
nervous system. *See also* brain; EEG (electroencephalography); neuromodulation
   about, 59–72, *60*
   electrical activity, 70–71, 178–179, 183
neuromodulation, 51, 96–97, 187–193
neurons
   about, 70–71, *72*
   and EEG recordings, 87, 88–89
neuropsychological evaluation, 195, 219, 246

neurotransmitters, 71, 178, 183
nonmotor signs and symptoms, 33–34, 35–36, *36,* 37–38, 39, 66
non-pharmaceutical treatments, 50, 51, 182–198

O
obesity, 227
obsessive-compulsive disorder (OCD), 230–231
occipital lobe, 63, *64,* 65
oppositional defiant disorder (ODD), 230
osteoporosis, 225

P
parents/caregivers
    and antiseizure medications, 168–169, 173–176
    and developmental milestones, 218
    and family-centered care, 52, 249
parietal lobe, 63, *64,* 65. *See also* somatosensory cortex
paroxysmal movement disorders, 226–227
peripheral nervous system, *60*
person-centered care, 52, 249–250
PET (positron emission tomography), 194
pharmaceutical treatments, 50, 51, 168–181, *172, 177*
physical activity, 240
pilot's license, 246
polytherapy, 51, 169–170
postictal phase of seizure, 42, *42,* 92
pregnancy, 171, 253–255
preictal phase of seizure, 41, *42,* 92
prolactin levels, 109
provoked seizures, 7–9, 28–29, *29*. *See also* reflex seizures
psychogenic nonepileptic seizures, 20
psychosis, 231

R
randomized controlled trial (RCT), 291–292
reading epilepsy, 7, 158
reflex epilepsy syndromes, 7, 157–158
reflex seizures, 4, 7. *See also* provoked seizures
remission, 49, 167

research
    and evidence-based medicine, 52, 206, 289–290
    getting involved in, 293–295
    types of study design, 290–293
responsive neurostimulation (RNS), *190,* 190–191
Rett syndrome, 221
risk factors, for epilepsy or seizures, 10
risky activities, 238–244

S
scuba diving, 246
seizure clusters, 165, 176, *177*
seizure diary, 96
seizure mimics, 15–21, *21*
seizure onset zone
    classification, 31–32, *32*
    and EEGs, 86–87
    identifying, 39, 63, 66
    neuropsychological evaluation, 195
    presurgical imaging, 193–194
seizure rescue medications, 171–173, 175–176, *177*
seizures. *See also* epilepsy
    about, 3–5, 71
    associated with lobes of cerebral cortex, 63, *65*
    causes and risk factors, 7–10
    classification, 31–40, *32, 33, 36, 38, 39, 40*
    control of, 49, 164 (*see also* antiseizure medications)
    danger from, 49–50, 165–166
    detecting and recording, 95–99, *97*
    differential diagnosis, 15–21, *21*
    first aid, 12–14, *13*
    freedom from, 49, 164–165
    and heart arrythmia, 85
    phases, 41–42, 92–93, *93, 94*
    prevalence, 10–11
    recurrence, 29–30
    triggers, 74, 80–81
seizure threshold, 73–74, 207
self-limited epilepsy syndromes, 142–143
self-limited focal epilepsy syndromes, 149–150
sensory symptoms, 35
shared decision-making, 52

side effects, adverse
  about, 168
  antiseizure medication, 171, 179–180, 206, 213, 225, 231
  herbal supplements, 207
  hyperbaric oxygen therapy, 207
  ketogenic diet, 185, 186
  medical cannabis, 202
  neuromodulation, 189, 191, 192
  steroids, 200
  surgery, 197–198
sleep disorders, 221
somatosensory cortex, 66, 67
somatosensory symptoms, 35, 66
sports, and epilepsy, 236, 240–244, *241, 242–243*
startle epilepsy, 7
status epilepticus, 49, 165, 166, 176, *177*
stereotactic radiosurgery, 197
steroids, 51, 199–200
structural epilepsy, 45, 106, 123–124
Sturge-Weber syndrome, 146
SUDEP (sudden unexpected death in epilepsy), 49, 53–54, 166
suicidality, 180, 230
surgery, for epilepsy, 51, 193–198
swimming, 244
syncope, 20
systematic review, 291

T
Takotsubo syndrome (TTS), 225
temporal lobe, 63, *64,* 65, 67, 68, *69*
temporal lobectomy, 195
tic disorders, 231
Todd's paralysis, 42
tonic-clonic movements, 37
tonic movements, 34–35, 37
toxicology screen, 110
transition from childhood to adulthood, 52, 249–250, *251, 252*
tuberous sclerosis complex, 221
tumors, 123–124

U
unknown epilepsy, 45, 133
unknown onset seizures, 32, 38–39, *39, 40*
unprovoked seizures, 9, 28–29, *29. See also* epilepsy

V
vagus nerve stimulation (VNS), 187–190, *188*
video EEG (VEEG), 79, 193–194. *See also* electroencephalography (EEG)
vitamins, 51, 200–201, 225

W
Wernicke's area, 67, *68*